PLASTIC SURGERY

Recent Titles in
Health and Medical Issues Today

Organ Transplantation
David Petechuk

Alternative Medicine
Christine A. Larson

Gene Therapy
Evelyn B. Kelly

Sports Medicine
Jennifer L. Minigh

Nutrition
Sharon Zoumbaris

HIV/AIDS
Kathy S. Stolley and John E. Glass

Medical Imaging
Harry LeVine, III

Medicare
Jennie Jacobs Kronenfeld

Illicit Drugs
Richard E. Isralowitz and Peter L. Myers

Animal-Assisted Therapy
Donald Altschiller

Alcohol
Peter L. Myers and Richard E. Isralowitz

Geriatrics
Carol Leth Stone

PLASTIC SURGERY

Lana Thompson

Health and Medical Issues Today

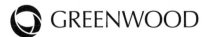 GREENWOOD

AN IMPRINT OF ABC-CLIO, LLC
Santa Barbara, California • Denver, Colorado • Oxford, England

Library of Congress Cataloging-in-Publication Data

Thompson, Lana.
    Plastic surgery / Lana Thompson.
        p. ; cm. — (Health and medical issues today)
    Includes bibliographical references and index.
    ISBN 978-0-313-37568-2 (hardback : alk. paper) —
    ISBN 978-0-313-37569-9 (eISBN)
    I. Title.   II. Series: Health and medical issues today.
    [DNLM: 1. Surgery, Plastic—history.   2. Reconstructive Surgical
Procedures—history.   3. Reconstructive Surgical Procedures—methods.
4. Surgery, Plastic—trends. WO 11.1]
    617.9'52—dc23   2011035547

ISBN: 978-0-313-37568-2
EISBN: 978-0-313-37569-9

16   15   14   13   12   1   2   3   4   5

This book is also available on the World Wide Web as an eBook.
Visit www.abc-clio.com for details.

Greenwood
An Imprint of ABC-CLIO, LLC

ABC-CLIO, LLC
130 Cremona Drive, P.O. Box 1911
Santa Barbara, California 93116-1911

This book is printed on acid-free paper ∞

Manufactured in the United States of America

Contents

SERIES FOREWORD

Every day, the public is bombarded with information on developments in medicine and health care. Whether it is on the latest techniques in treatment or research, or on concerns over public health threats, this information directly affects the lives of people more than almost any other issue. Although there are many sources for understanding these topics—from Web sites and blogs to newspapers and magazines—students and ordinary citizens often need one resource that makes sense of the complex health and medical issues affecting their daily lives.

The Health and Medical Issues Today series provides just such a one-stop resource for obtaining a solid overview of the most controversial areas of health care in the 21st century. Each volume addresses one topic and provides a balanced summary of what is known. These volumes provide an excellent first step for students and lay people interested in understanding how health care works in our society today.

Each volume is broken into several sections to provide readers and researchers with easy access to the information they need:

Section I provides overview chapters on background information—including chapters on such areas as the historical, scientific, medical, social, and legal issues involved—that a citizen needs to intelligently understand the topic.

Section II provides capsule examinations of the most heated contemporary issues and debates, and analyzes in a balanced manner the viewpoints held by various advocates in the debates.

Section III provides a selection of reference material, such as annotated primary source documents, a timeline of important events, and a directory of organizations that serve as the best next step in learning about the topic at hand.

The Health and Medical Issues Today series strives to provide readers with all the information needed to begin making sense of some of the most important debates going on in the world today. The series includes volumes on such topics as stem-cell research, obesity, gene therapy, alternative medicine, organ transplantation, mental health, and more.

SECTION I

Introduction

When one thinks about plastic surgery, one might imagine a woman, attractive, ageless, self-confident, perhaps somewhat artificial, who has been "made over" by a doctor. She has gone to great pains to escape what she interprets as the ravages of age, to mask wrinkles, fatty deposits, sagging flesh, or some other "imperfection." Advertisements for plastic surgery often depict the patient as female and the doctor as male, paternalistic and sympathetic. The plastic surgeon's waiting room would be appointed in elegant furnishings to suggest luxury: leather couches and chairs, thick glass coffee tables with fashion magazines and images of beautiful people. On one wall, patient information brochures and booklets on every imaginable procedure would be neatly stacked on a Lucite rack. These publications, sanctioned by the American Board of Plastic Surgeons, would have titles such as Blepharoplasty, Abdominoplasty, Rhinoplasty, Liposuction, Botox, and Restylan, to mention a few. The women in the pictures would be young and attractive. However, this envisions only one type of plastic surgery, the popularized cosmetic or esthetic plastic surgery, the answer to fantasized ideals. In reality, plastic surgery is much more than fixing the signs of age or desperately seeking perfection. It is a medical specialty that arose from the need to undo the violence perpetrated by humans against other humans, in fights, battles, wars or nuclear disasters.

Some of the early damage to facial features was extreme corporal punishment in the form of nose amputations for sinners, men who had committed adultery. Those men were stigmatized for life unless they could get some kind of correction. Some of the first surgical procedures were developed to restore noses. A long period of progress in general surgery and anatomy had to take place before plastic surgery could branch out. Fortunately, barber-surgeons were available to practice surgery in a world that was otherwise closed to the only educated class. Barber-surgeons shaved the monks because the brothers were forbidden to "shed blood." With that, barbers took over other bodily tasks involving penetrating the skin. Competing with barber-surgeons for patients were charlatans, mountebanks, and other self-taught individuals. This both heightened and made more urgent the need for professionalism. Guilds were established and the first medical associations formed. However, a series of disruptions to titled medical people continued until barber-surgeons demanded to be referred to as surgeons and remove the "barber" from their names. Culture wars ensued and resulted in two categories of medical people: The Royal College of Surgeons and The Royal College of Physicians. This distinction between physicians and surgeons exists in the United States today, although it is no longer "royal."

The first plastic surgery images are of a Gasparo Tagliacozzi (1546–1599) patient whose elbow is lifted near his face, supported by a brace, illustrating an early graft procedure for a facial wound. During the Renaissance and early modern periods, plastic surgery's original mission was to restore function to faces that had been maimed by a variety of traumas: deliberate amputations, fire, crushing injuries, and when genetic anomalies required repair of vital tissues. Successive wars created greater challenges, due to the increasingly destructive technology involved. Great medical advances of the mid-19th century, including the development of anesthesia and antibiotics, gave surgeons more time to keep a patient unconscious during surgery and to prevent post-operative infections. This enabled a great leap forward in the practice of surgery.

The First World War led to the development of different types of flaps to be used for reconstruction. When defects could not be corrected, strange prostheses were created to hide the horrific appearance of burn scars or wounds that would not heal. Gaston Leroux's (1868–1927) character, Erik, in *The Phantom of the Opera,* was allegedly born without a nose and was, therefore, so hideous that his mother fashioned him a mask immediately after he was born. "He asked only to be 'some one,' like everybody else. But he was too ugly! And he had to hide his genius . . . when, with an ordinary face, he would have been one of the most distinguished of mankind!" (Leroux 2008, 220). That desire to "normalize" patients is one of the greatest missions of the medical profession and grew more extreme, if not distorted, with the progression of plastic surgery as a specialty. One might think that everyone would agree to the importance of normalization; however, many of the controversies involved in plastic surgery confront differences in opinions regarding such an assumption.

In the 21st century, these "normalization" alterations morphed to include liposuction (to restore a slim body to one that has become fat), rhinoplasty (to change a nose that perhaps stigmatizes an individual because of ethnic concerns), Botox (to remove wrinkles and signs of age), collagen injections, and breast augmentation (to restore youth or enhance beauty).

Thus, the majority of information about plastic surgery is associated with some kind of "magical" process whereby one's looks are improved to such an extent that they transcend the average or normal. But there is more to plastic surgery than esthetics or cosmetic enhancement. Plastic surgery is performed to correct a congenital or birth defect that interferes with function or to repair a wound caused by a traumatic event.

REFERENCE

Leroux, Gaston. 2008. *The Phantom of the Opera.* Project Gutenberg.

CHAPTER 1

History

Plastic surgery's early history is documented in Indian and Egyptian writings. Although the translations differ, there are common threads that connect those surgical techniques that eventually evolved into a medical specialty. There is a fuzzy distinction between the scriptures of gods and goddesses and those of actual healers because all healing was originally attributed to mythological characters. Some healers, such as medicine men, wise women, curanderos, shamans, and other designated healers in a society, said they received divine information from the gods. Whether these early documents represent the teachings of a celestial being or a real person, the information exists.

One theme featured throughout the early history of plastic surgery is its close association with social needs and acceptance. Since humans evolved to walk in upright positions, the face evolved to have less hair, a greater distance between the eyes, and an elaborate network of muscles and nerves that serve to express emotion. Because the face is so important in social interaction, any defect or unusual feature communicates significant nonverbal information. Thus, fixing and restoring the face is of primary importance to humans.

The progress in saving lives and restoring tissues that early surgeons achieved depended on both an awareness of the social value of the human face and the ability to use nonhuman animals for experimentation on tissue healing and grafting. Although the knowledge and techniques of the early practitioners appear unsophisticated compared with modern surgeons, the present-day results that appear miraculous were only made possible by standing on the shoulders of these early giants.

EGYPT

The beginnings of plastic surgery are recorded in ancient Egyptian and Indian writings. The Edwin Smith Papyrus (circa 3000–2200 BCE) from

India, translated by James Henry Breasted in the early 20th century, described 48 surgical cases. Within these case studies, we found instructions for wound healing using sutures, the treatment of mandibular and nasal fractures, and care for postoperative and traumatic hematoma. There is text of three cases regarding broken noses in which the physician is instructed by Imhotep, a master sculpture and healer, who is later elevated to the status of a god. Imhotep advises the physician to force the broken nose to fall so that it is in place, and then clean out the inside of both nostrils with swabs of linen. After the bleeding stops and the blood clots come out, the physician is to insert two plugs of linen saturated with grease. On the outside of the nose, he is to place stiff rolls of linen or thin wooden splints padded with linen alongside of the nose to maintain its normal shape. Later writings of Pliny the Elder (23–79 CE) indicated that the Egyptians used powdered marble mixed with vinegar to create a counter-irritant which acted as a local anesthetic, though there is nothing in Imhotep's advice on the surgical narrative to confirm that.

INDIA

In northern India, around 500 BCE, the Koomas developed the method of transferring skin from the forehead and/or cheek to the nose. One man, *Sushruta* is referred to as the father of plastic surgery. The name, *Sushruta,* means "the one who is well heard," or "the one who has thoroughly learned by hearing" and the *Sushruta Samhita* is the text that has been handed down from ancient Indian medical practitioners. Sushruta's greatest contributions were his descriptions of how to repair nasal defects using: sliding grafts (release of the skin for covering small defects), rotational grafts (rotation of the flaps to compensate for partial loss of tissue), and pedicle grafts (flaps to cover a complete loss of skin from an area).

"When a man's nose has been cut off or destroyed, the physician takes a leaf of a creeper, long and broad enough to be of the size of destroyed parts. He places it on the patient's cheek and slices off of his cheek a piece of skin of the same size (in such manner that the skin at one end remains attached to the cheek). After scarifying the stump of the nose with a knife, he wraps the piece of skin from the cheek carefully all around it and sews it at the edges (using the huge heads of ants). Then he inserts two thin pipes in the nose (in the position of nostrils) to facilitate respiration and prevent flesh from collapsing. The adhesioned part is then dusted with powders of Pattanga, Yashtimadhukam, and Rasanjana pulverized together. The nose is then enveloped in Karpasa cotton and several times sprinkled over with the refined oil of pure sesame. When the healing is complete and parts have united, the connection with the cheek is removed"

(Sorta-Bijalac and Mazur 2007, 707). This method of repair is referred to as "the Indian method of rhinoplasty."

In India, amputation of the nose was a common and well-documented punishment. Bands of invaders from enemy territories would terrorize settled groups by mutilating the faces of the vanquished as a lasting mark of the victors' power. One creation myth tells how Rama, a Hindu god, amputated women's noses as an example of acceptable earthly behavior for men to inflict on those women who do not conform to their husband's rules. Therefore, the nose had a symbolic significance: it represented one's physical integrity and reputation. Being prominent on the face, it was constantly exposed to scrutiny. Once a person's nose was amputated or damaged, their status changed and the person was no longer respected. Often, the shame and humiliation was so great that those without a nose became reclusive or suicidal. The pejorative term, *al-Majdū*, referred to a person whose nose has been cut off. There is evidence that a group known as the Isma'ilis in India practiced nose amputation as punishment well into the 12th century.

GREECE

Independently, Hippocrates (460–375 BCE), a Greek physician, recommended that a hollow wooden tube (*shalak*) be put in each nostril to maintain the nostril's former, normal shape until the broken bones healed, as written in his book *Mochlicon*. Anthyllus, in the second century, recommended that a dressing made from cotton or silk should be used to fill the nostrils and not be removed until the nose healed. Perhaps he intended to also write that the dressing should be changed every few days.

ROME

In Rome, plastic surgery is documented extensively in the writings of Aulus Cornelius Celsus (50–25 BCE) in *De Medicina Octo Libri* (*The Eight Books of Medicine*). These books are written in Latin, translated from the Greek. Evidently, Celsus had a great deal of experience repairing fractured faces, because he wrote about correcting a misshapen nose, repairing cartilage in the ear, using flaps to repair defects in the lower lip, and repairing ears damaged by heavy earrings or other mutilations. Book VII also tells how to create a prepuce on a penis where the "glans is bare and the man wishes for the look of the thing to have it covered," as well as performing a circumcision where a phimosis exists (Celsus Book VII. 24. 1–25. c). When Emperor Justinian II was overthrown, his usurpers mutilated his nose as a way to humiliate and prevent him from ever regaining his political status. Using a Celsus technique, an early practitioner performed a flap procedure to restore Emperor Justinian II's appearance. The statue known as *Rhinometus* is believed to be a sculpture of him, and upon close inspection, the surgical defect can be seen.

Celsus's other specialty was restoring the prepuce of circumcised Jewish men to hide their religious origins, in the event they sought political office. He recorded two procedures: one that stretched the foreskin, incised the skin at the root of the penis and banded it until it remained in place, and a second procedure that took the skin at the corona of the penis, separated it from the *corpora cavernosa*, pulled it over the glans, and fixed it there with sutures. Evidently, if one wanted to rise in politics, or participate in Greek athletic games, one could not be Jewish or show evidence of their Jewishness through a circumcised penis.

It is puzzling that congenital defects such as cleft palate and harelip are missing from the ancient medical literature of Italy and Greece, or are not as frequently found as in Egypt or India. Perhaps the practice of infanticide, coupled with the belief that some sort of evil caused the anomalies, account for its absence. One statuette found in Corinth, dating from 700–300 BCE, is of a clown with a harelip. However, there are writings of Galen's that describe the use of local flaps to repair lip defects other than harelip.

When Rome fell, ongoing progress came to a standstill in improving plastic surgery techniques and applications. Other than the writings of Byzantine physician Paul of Aegina (Paulus Aegineta), the historical record lacks continuity. Paul of Aegina (625–690 CE) validated the importance of reshaping and realigning broken nasal bones to retain the nose's former shape. He preached urgency by noting that if the bones were not aligned by the tenth day, they would mend in the broken position. He recommended fashioning two wedge-like tents formed from a twisted linen rag, and putting one on the side of each nostril (Santoni-Rugiu and Sykes 2007, 169). Paul designed and used special scalpels for ectropion, entropian, and lagophthalmos. Aegina had an interest in facial wrinkles, as well. He advised the patient to rub the skin with a tablet made from the shavings of ivory, fish gelatin, and frankincense in order to counter the effects of aging.

MEDIEVAL PERIOD

The conquest of India in the 10th century by various Islamic groups created a "knowledge gateway" that allowed the flow of information between East and West. The Arabic culture had much to offer Europe, particularly regarding the surgical techniques of the ancients. For approximately 400 years, this cross-cultural knowledge sharing thrived, but, unfortunately, few new procedures were practiced or medical compounds developed.

A variety of factors delayed the progress in medicine and surgery. In addition to the lack of formal secular institutions of learning, there were religious and cultural aversions to learning about anatomy. Further Pope Innocent III (1160–1216) banned all surgical procedures because the Church abhorred the shedding of blood. This maxim persisted throughout Europe and was used to deny both anatomical dissection and surgery. The sole exception involved cases of suspicious deaths, where poisoning was suspected, within monasteries. In 1248, the Council of Le Mans forbid monks to perform surgery and Pope Boniface VIII (1235–1303) issued the decretal prohibiting crusaders from carrying back the bones of those who had died while traveling to foreign lands. This was broadly interpreted as a proscription against dissection and autopsy; thus, the academic pursuit of knowledge was interrupted because of a misunderstanding. The outcome was the perpetuation of ignorance regarding human anatomy and physiology, and the practice of medicine devolved and fell into the hands of the uneducated barber-surgeons, mountebanks, herbalists, apothecaries, midwives, and charlatans. This is not to say that all barber-surgeons or midwives were poorly trained, but there were no regulated standards for education or training. Over a period of 500 years, various societal changes such as a population shift from rural to urban, the emergence of a middle class, and nonsecular education opportunities at academic institutions lead to a medical profession with strict guidelines for specialty training.

NEW WORLD

The New World, by contrast, particularly the pre-Columbian cultures of West Mexico and Coastal Peru, produced a great number of statuettes depicting congenital anomalies, including harelip, cleft palate, phocomelia, lack of ear cartilage, and lobster-claw hands. Those cultures, rather than scorn the anomalous, believed that dwarves, epileptics, or individuals who fell outside of the norm were special or gifted. Oftentimes, a physical anomaly was seen as a sign that the person was a shaman (a gifted individual with the ability to heal others). It is probable that any individual who survived infancy and childhood with a cleft palate was regarded as a sage or person in touch with the spiritual world, and would not have undergone any kind of physical modification. In certain cultures, one had to be visibly or psychologically different if one wished to be a healer.

RENAISSANCE

Barber-Surgeons

The barbers who shaved monks were trained to perform blood-letting (phlebotomy), a common form of medical treatment used to treat a variety of illnesses. In England in 1462, barbers were authorized to practice surgery, and in 1540 surgeons and barbers were united by a royal decree that grouped them into the United Barber-Surgeons Company. In France, barbers were distinguished from "real" surgeons and known as "wound" surgeons. Barber-surgeons treated the horrific bodily damage caused by gunpowder, then a new invention, and were often acquainted with such wounds. Despite their growing utility, they were still considered irregular practitioners.

Medicine becomes Professionalized

The practice of medicine changed from sacred to secular in Europe as universities were built. This was the birth of professionalized medicine. During that period when barber surgeons, physicians, and practitioners of professionalized medicine competed for patients, training was variable at best. Knowledge about treatment or surgeries was passed from father to son and that experience remained at a premium. Henry de Mondeville (1260–1320) wrote that anatomical knowledge was essential for anyone who practiced surgery and bodies of deceased humans rather than animals were necessary for practice. Despite his advocacy for learning, the body was still regarded as something not to be observed. Social taboos, particularly about women's bodies, prevented widespread information, autopsy or dissection of females. Those who were fortunate enough to see a human dissection were rare.

Fifteenth Century

For almost 300 years, the plastic surgical techniques of India, Greece, and Italy remained at a standstill. This all changed around 1442 when the Sicilian barber-surgeon Gustavo Branca was said to have used the Indian method for making local flaps to restore noses. He passed this technique down to his son, Antonio, who then experimented with "distant" or "delayed flaps," using a donor site from the upper arm. This became known as the Italian method; that is, to use a pedicled skin flap from the arm. Using skin from the arm instead of the face quickly became the norm cosmetically because it left fewer scars on the face. The son, Antonio, shared this technique with another family of barber-surgeons, the Vianeos brothers in Calabria, and Alessandro Benedetti (1460–1525), a professor of surgery in Padua. Neither Brancas nor the Vianeos published their findings, because they preferred to keep their information to themselves rather than invite competition. Benedetti reported it in 1502 in his book, *Anatomice, Sive Historia Corporis Humani* (*Anatomy or the History of the Human Body*), but opinions differ as to whether he actually performed the surgery. His writings indicate a certain amount of experience, because he cautions the patient with the newly constructed nose that it is quite fragile, and writing that during winter, one should not hold one's nose because it might detach from the face and remain in the hand. Although the 16th-century surgeon Tagliacozzi is generally credited with this Italian method, parts of his manuscript are identical to Benedetti's work.

In Germany around 1460, a Bavarian army surgeon, Henrich von Pfolspeundt, was working with a similar technique using skin from the arm. He would cut a flap from the bicep, sew it onto the nose to cover the defect, and then bandage the arm to the head. After eight to ten days of healing, he would divide the pedicle and form the rest of the nose. His work, *Wund-Arznei* (*Wound Doctor*), cautioned the reader, "If one comes to you

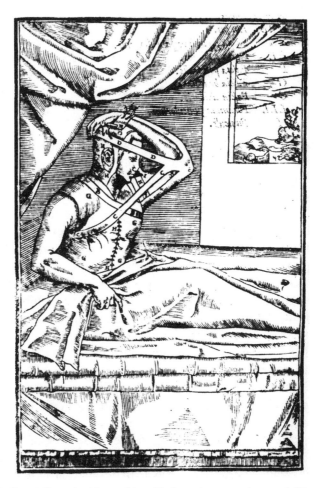

Gaspare Tagliacozzi's method for grafting skin from the arm to the nose is illustrated in this 16th-century woodcut. (National Library of Medicine)

with a cut off nose, let no one watch and make him swear to tell nobody how you cured him."[1]

Sixteenth Century

When the Bolognese surgeon and doctor of medicine Leonardo Fioravanti (1517–1588) returned from the Crusades, he stopped in Calabria to visit the Vianeos brothers, under the guise of an interested traveler, not revealing his profession. He observed several surgeries and after returning home, published *Il Tesoro della Vita Umana* (The Treasure of Life), outlining what he had learned by watching the Vianeos brothers (Santoni-Rugiu and Mazzola 1997, 750). His contemporary, Gaspare Tagliacozzi (1545–1599), a professor of anatomy and surgery at the University of Bologna, studied the information and developed the technique that became the standard pedicled flap. This was the basis for the development of modern plastic surgery. His 1597 book *De Curtorum Chirurgia per insitionem* (which roughly translates to "surgery using grafting") was more than 100 pages long and replete with magnificent illustrations and detailed descriptions of such techniques. The book was criticized by two of his contemporaries, Ambröise Paré (1510–1590) and Gabriele Fallopius, because he was allegedly interfering with the work of God.[2] Paré, the master barber-surgeon, was best known for putting an end to the use of boiling oil for gunshot wounds, for the use of sutures instead of cauterization after amputation, and for the design of elegant and complex prostheses for the wounded. His prosthetic hands were made from complex, ornate-looking interlocking leaves of metal. Despite the fact that he was well aware of the psychological damage that deformities, scars, and blemishes could inflict on an individual, he was critical of what his contemporaries did to alter the appearance of others.

The caveat that "man" should not meddle with the work of God has been invoked throughout the history of medicine. The prohibition against endorsing medical progress usually accompanies a radical change, such as the discovery of a "miracle drug," a way to prevent illness, or a surgical procedure that restores functionality previously believed to be impossible. The opposition to anesthesia was justified because pain, particularly pain in childbirth, was thought to be God's punishment for original sin. Vaccines, antibiotics, and treatment for venereal disease were each met with resistance, because of the belief that disease was a consequence of some moral infringement or punishment for sacrilege. Because of the nature of the outcomes, plastic surgery, in particular, has always been subject to a great deal of scrutiny because of the boundaries that separate necessity or reconstruction, and esthetics or cosmesis. Fortunately, the history of medicine has yielded to progress rather than superstition and allowed these inventions and discoveries, but sometimes not soon enough. Interestingly, neither Paré nor Fallopius considered their own work as meddling.

EIGHTEENTH AND NINETEENTH CENTURY

For another 200 years, a period of dormancy slowed the progress of plastic surgery.[3] For example, in 1788, the Paris Faculty forbade any facial repairing, even though some reconstructive surgery was being performed in the British Isles. In Chelsea, England, the surgeon, Joseph Constantine Carpue (1764–1846) read of another British surgeon who had reconstructed an Indian's nose in India by using a triangular forehead flap. The author of the letter was unknown, identified only by the initials, B. L. Like many an urban myth, his narration began with the typical "A friend knew of a . . ." and went on to describe Cowasjee, a bullock driver, who was made a prisoner and had his nose and one of his hands cut off under the orders of Tippoo Sultan. The "friend" did not see the surgery but he knew two medical gentlemen who had seen an operation to restore a nose performed using skin from the forehead. The document was in the form of a letter to the editor in *Gentlemen's Quarterly* (1794). It was the first time that information about rhinoplasties in India was shared with readers in Europe. Carpue was inspired to try the technique described in the letter but wanted more information, so he first sought people who had traveled to India and asked if any of them had heard of such an operation. One employee of the East India Company told him that such an operation is performed in only 30 minutes. Carpue was intrigued but unable to find out anything more. He continued to teach and write, but he remained intent on learning how to perform this surgery. He recommended it to his pupils, but still had no experience in performing it. As fortune would have it, in 1814, an army officer with a mutilated nose approached him and said that he had heard of Carpue's reputation in Gibraltar regarding an operation to restore a "lost nose." The officer had been in Egypt and been afflicted with a liver complaint. During the 14 years following, he had been treated with mercury so many times that his nose no longer had a septum, the anterior part of the cartilage, and a small portion of the alae (wings), and had begun to slough off. Carpue consented to do the surgery, but warned the officer that he had not yet performed such an operation. The patient was otherwise healthy, but to be sure, Carpue made some experimental incisions at the base of the nose to determine if the tissues would heal correctly. Satisfied that the tissues were healthy enough for surgery, he practiced on a series of corpses until he was confident enough to try it on a living being. One final time, he performed the procedure on a cadaver, this time in an operating theater in front of his surgeon friends and pupils. Reassured by his peers, he proceeded to undertake the "live" surgery. Using a wax model as a template for the graft, he laid the template on the man's forehead and drew the outline on the skin. The patient was not anesthetized and stated that he hoped to "behave like a man" (Carpue 1816, 85). Afterward, he said that the procedure was extremely painful, but he knew there was no use in complaining. After the dressings were applied, he felt nothing. Carpue had been attentive to every detail of B. L.'s letter, even heating the operating room to match what he imagined as the temperature and humidity of Indian continent. His surgery on the officer was successful, as evidenced by the exclamation of a fellow officer's response, "My God, there is a nose." His second patient, Captain Latham, had been fighting at the battle of Albuera in Spain when he lost an arm to a saber cut, before receiving additional wounds to his nose and cheek. Latham's appearance was badly compromised, he was plagued by colds, and the exposed skin was often inflamed. Instead of a more symmetrical repair, he opted for a procedure that removed less healthy tissue, limited the scar to the middle of his nose, yet only repaired one half of his nose. He approached Carpue and asked him if he could restore his nose through surgery. Using a pedicled flap taken from the forehead, Carpue reconstructed the man's nose in two stages. After the forehead healed, he made another incision in the "new" nose and made it fit into the "old" nose, securing the tissues with silver pins and a suture. Both reports were published in the monograph, *An Account of Two Successful Operations for Restoring a Lost Nose from the Integuments of the Forehead.*

Johann Friedrich Dieffenbach (1794–1847), a physician in Berlin, read Carpue's 1816 publication and performed a number of rhinoplasties, in addition to a variety of other surgeries. He completed successful skin transplants using leeches to restore circulation, repaired tendons, and preformed surgery to correct crossed eyes. Ahead of his time, his initial thesis described a hair-transplant surgery that he performed (*Regeneratione Transplantatione, Dissertatio inauguralis* [Initial dissertation, transplant regeneration]). Dieffenbach was interested in the psychological component of physiological disorders, such as stuttering and blinking. He observed after surgery to repair a deviated septum that, in addition to the physical improvement to his patient's appearance, the patient's self esteem also improved. This aspect of medicine was to become a crucial concern and controversy regarding justification for performing certain plastic procedures. He used the term "beauty surgery," meaning cosmetic, to differentiate it from "real" surgery, meaning corrective procedures. His experience seeing trauma as a young man in the war affected him so much that he decided to become a surgeon. Referred to as the "father of plastic surgery," he was the first surgeon to successfully close a hard-palate cleft.

Eighteenth-century plastic surgeons continued to investigate skin grafts, because such procedures were necessary to replace the tissue damaged by burns and wounds. Since the reasons for tissue rejection were unknown, the results were often puzzling. Why did some grafts work and others not? Giuseppe Baronio (1758–1814) took large strips of skin from a ram and transplanted each to the other side of the animal's body. He knew that a certain amount of tissue shrinkage occurred at the margins and accounted for that by putting tape along the edges. Healing did occur in both sites. Afterward, he cut into each transplanted piece to make certain that vascularization (blood supply) had occurred, and it had. Baronio continued to experiment with a variety of animals: cows, goats, horses, and dogs and received positive results. But, like the innovators before him, his peers either dismissed his optimism or ignored his accounts when he tried to share his results with them. Undaunted, Baronio continued to maintain records and manipulate variables, such as time intervals between procedures and surgical conditions, to learn which factors guaranteed the best healing. Although grafts worked when transplanted from one area of the body to another in the same animal, they were rejected when transplanted from animal to animal. Second to Tagliacozzi, Baronio represented the succeeding milestone in the history of plastic surgery. Although he published a book about a new concept—the union of the two tissues and the necessity of a certain amount of inflammation—his work continued to be ignored. The *vital principle* that he discovered that allowed two injured parts to grow together became known as *fibrin*. Perhaps the language barrier prevented Baronio's acceptance, because he wrote in Italian (in 1804), and it was not translated into German until 1819. Or perhaps surgeons were more interested in using flaps, restoring noses the Indian way, instead of performing skin grafts.

Notes

1. There was also a German surgeon, Heinrich von Pfalzpaint, who is known to have performed rhinoplasties.

2. So incensed were Paré and others over Tagliacozzi's work that his remains were exhumed from the convent where they were interred in consecrated ground, and reburied in non-consecrated land.

3. In 1907, a description of an Indian rhinoplasty was discovered. Allegedly written in the 17th century by the Italian adventurer, Nicolò Manuzzi (a.k.a. Manucci, 1639–1717), its veracity is questionable.

References

Carpue, J.C. 1816. *An Account of two successful operations for restoring a lost nose from the integuments of the forehead, in the cases of two officers of his majesty's army; to which are prefixed, historical and physiological remarks on the nasal operation; including descriptions of the Indian and Italian methods.* London: Longman, Hurst, Rees, Orme and Brown.

Santoni-Rugiu, Paolo, and R. Mazzola. 1997. "Leonardo Fioravanti (1517–1588): A Barber-Surgeon Who Influenced the Development of Reconstructive Surgery." *Plastic and Reconstructive Surgery* 99: 570–75.

Santoni-Rugiu, Paolo, and Phillip Sykes. 2007. *A History of Plastic Surgery.* New York: Springer Verlag.

Sorta-Bijalac, Iva, and Amir Mazur. 2007. "The Nose between Ethics and Aesthetics: Sushruta's Legacy." *Otolaryngology—Head and Neck Surgery* 137: 707–10.

CHAPTER 2

Indications and Types of Treatment

Other than genetic anomalies and birth defects, historically the most severe traumatic events that required surgery were burns from gunshot wounds or fires, wounds that extended beyond the skin—into muscle and ligament, cancers, and chronic festering infections that destroyed tissue and refused to heal. To treat those injuries, doctors developed a variety of grafts, flaps, and implants. Initially, plastic surgery was a small specialty primarily devoted to reestablishing normal function in children with developmental defects or to repair wounds that required grafts. However, in between the two World Wars, plastic surgery developed into a huge specialty. The specialty to repair the errors of inheritance or damage sustained by the human body has undergone many changes in technique, training, and technology. In addition to these emergent medical necessities, cosmetic or esthetic plastic surgery developed into a specialty within a specialty.

DEFORMITIES FROM BURNS

Burns have been one of the most complex challenges facing plastic surgeons. Prior to Ambröise Paré, treatments exacerbated the problems of pain, infection, and scarring. Pouring boiling oil on open wounds, the traditional medieval treatment, hardly seems logical, yet that was the practice until Paré abandoned it in favor of simple dressings. Burn victims lose fluid and become dehydrated because their body's surface area is no longer protected by skin and cannot prevent or limit fluid loss. Infection occurs because skin, the first line of defense, has been destroyed. After the burn begins to heal, other problems confront the patient. Functionally, there is a loss of sensation in the scar tissue and restriction of motion. The scar is incised so that the adhesions that restrict movement can be broken to allow greater flexibility. In the case of facial burns, the horrible scarring that causes major deformities was a complex problem, with both psychological and physical aspects.

The physician Thomas Dent Mütter (1811–1859) operated on a woman who as a child was scarred by burning after her clothes were set on fire. Her face, throat, and chest were burned in such a way that the scar tissue impeded movement of her head to the left and backwards. She was also unable to close her mouth for more than a few seconds and her right eye was affected so that it was drawn down and would close completely if she moved her head to the right. Mütter published his results from treating her, as well as three others cases, in his monograph *Cases of Deformity from Burns, Successfully Treated by Plastic Operations* (1843). This and many other publications documented a career devoted to caring for and restoring function to severely burned individuals. A sample of Mütter's monograph is reprinted in Section III, Appendix A, Document 1.

ADVANCEMENT FLAPS AND TUBE FLAPS

In France, Francois Chopart (1743–1795) worked with the skin from the chin to repair lower lip defects caused by cancer. Even though both Celsus and the Hindus had employed similar flaps, the French took credit for this type of advancement flap and named it *procédée du tiroir* (which loosely translates to "drawer procedure," because it made two parallel incisions under the chin). Others soon modified Chopart's technique. Charles Francois Lallemand (1790–1854) moved the base of the flap to below the chin, and this became known as the *advancement flap.* Later in 1828, Philibert Joseph Roux (1780–1854) wrote about a new method for operating on lip cancer using an undermined flap (*Mémoires sur le cancer des levres et sur une nouvelle methode operatoire* [Memoirs on lip cancer and on a new surgical method]).

J. Morgan and C. Viguerie, from Guy's Hospital in London, used Chopart's flap as a model and modified it in various ways (1829). They used a bipedicle (double pedicle, tube, or suitcase handle) flap. This is a skin flap that is created by making two parallel incisions and then rolling the created strip into a tube or handle. When the tube heals from its initial position, it is removed and used to correct a defect or create a missing mass of tissue, such as an ear lobe. Tubular flaps are a technique that has carried over from therapeutic to fashionable use. Modern body modification enthusiasts and punk rockers go to plastic surgeons to have bipedicle or tubular flaps created so that they can leave handle-like skin on their body and decorate the flap with distinctive jewelry.

One problem with the advancement flap is that it often healed with thickened folds that were unattractive and interfered with function. As often in the history of invention, two people (with no common connection other than their specialty) came up with a solution, independently yet at approximately the same time. So it was with Camille Bernard and Karl von Burow. Bernard gave a presentation to the Société de Chirurgie de Paris in 1852 in France. Von Burow (1809–1864) published a paper in England. Each advocated that a triangular piece of skin be removed from each side of the flap to facilitate its direction of growth. In France, the modification was called the *Burow–Bernard technique* and in England, *Burow's Triangle.*

In Germany, doctors experimented with other places on the face that would be amenable to plastic surgery. The area between the lip and the nose (*nasiolabal sulcus*) was ideal for certain lip flaps because the area

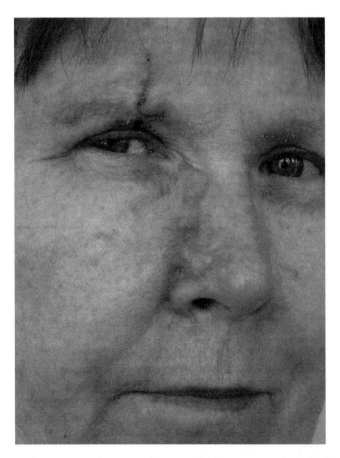

Moh's surgery has proven to be extremely successful in treatment of certain skin cancers because it leaves less facial scarring and removes only a minimum of tissue. (Courtesy of Marilyn Whittington)

healed well with sutures. Johan Karl Fricke (1790–1841) reconstructed an eyelid from the remaining skin around the patient's eye.

In 1817, Henry M. Dutrochet (1776–1847) described a new way that a nose could be repaired using a graft instead of a flap. The difference in the two procedures is that a flap depends on the surrounding or connecting tissue for blood supply and is attached to the defect; a graft is the introduction of a completely independent piece of tissue removed from another part of the body that gets its blood supply from the vessels near the defect. In Dutrochet's method, the patient's nose was restored with a piece of tissue taken from his buttock and was attached using adhesive plaster. Like Baronio, Dutrochet recognized the importance of preventing inflammation, so prior to removing the tissue for the graft, he used a stick to beat the buttock until it became red and swollen. By doing so, the blood vessels responded by allowing more blood to enter the area.

GRAFTS

The process of beating tissue to create a well-vascularized graft was termed *flagellation*. While appearing brutal, it prepares the tissue for adhering to new cells and became well accepted among surgeons performing grafts. In Germany, Christian Heinrich Bünger (1782–1842) operated on a woman's nose, using skin with flagellated fat pulled from her thigh. The graft was sewn onto the defect and, after three days, demonstrated viability and success.

In Erlangen, Germany, Carl Thiersch (1822–1895) worked with patients suffering skin cancer and demonstrated how epithelial cancer metastasized with malignant cells. Perhaps because of his interest in the inflammatory process, he found the positive aspect of this process: the self-proliferation of cells. When the donor site was pounded or flagellated, cells were stimulated to reproduce. Together with Louis Léopold Ollier (1830–1900) in Leipzig, Germany, Thiersch developed split-skin grafting. This procedure is known as Ollier–Thiersch graft, or the split-thickness graft. The new twist was the tissue was flagellation at both the transplant and the donor site. In London at Guy's Hospital, Sir Astley Cooper (1768–1841), an anatomist and surgeon best known for his work with vascular surgery, reported that he had successfully covered the stump of an amputated thumb with a graft from the detached thumb. The narrative is documented in his surgical essays in a collection of Underwood Lectures written in 1824, 1825, and 1827.

Antisepsis

A major risk with grafted material was the propensity for development of infections. Since no one kept accurate worldwide statistics regarding outcomes of graft procedures, failure rates can only be imagined. Antisepsis was barely accepted and sporadically practiced: sterile technique with masks, gloves, drapes, and clean instruments had yet become standard practice. Despite the statistics compiled by Ignaz Semmelweis in 1847 about the relationship of sepsis in recently deceased and childbed fever (i.e., the development of infections that led to the deaths of young women), his work was still not regarded as important. He had found that simple hand washing after leaving the morgue and before examining women in labor would prevent infection. Unfortunately, his colleagues would not accept the information (Magner 1922, 266; Lyons and Petrucelli 1987, 553). He lectured on the importance of cleaning pus and blood off any hand that would touch another patient, but the concept of "germ" had yet to be discovered or recognized. Semmelweis knew there was "something" that was transmitted from decomposed bodies to healthy ones, but that something was neither seen nor understood. It would be another 20 years before Joseph Lister (1827–1912) published his work on the treatment of wounds with carbolic acid (phenol), based on the principles of Pasteur's work with bacteria. Lister found that he could prevent the spread of necrosis by the application of a rag soaked in this chemical. He experimented with treating abscesses, compound fractures, and gangrene with antisepsis, and then hypothesized that if the most severe forms of wounds could heal using carbolic acid, so could incised wounds.

Neither infection nor tissue rejection were understood as reasons for failing grafts. Elie Metchnikoff (1845–1916), a Russian biologist, studied phagocytosis in lower animals and recognized that certain white blood cells destroyed foreign bodies in the bloodstream. His publications were met with initial rejection by the scientific community, because current belief was that white blood cells helped rather than hindered invading bacteria. Still, he persisted in studying the complex workings of the immune system and in 1908 shared the Nobel Prize with Paul Ehrlich for their work on immunity. The specific cells and organs that are responsible for preserving health of the individual were not known until the latter part of the 20th century, but Metchnikoff's early work helped physicians better understand the healing process. Paul Bert (1833–1886) was able to classify and identify states of success or failure in the process of grafting. In his doctoral thesis, he defined the concepts of *autograft* (grafting a tissue into a new position in the body of the same individual), *homograft* (allograft; a graft from one individual to another of the same species), and *heterograft* (xenograft; a graft from one species to another). He described the different success rates and noted that autografts were always more successful than the other two, although he could not explain why.

Christian Billroth (1829–1894) worked with burn patients and found that certain cells at the site of injury would form new tissue, called granulation tissue, as the wounds healed. The process, called *epithelialization*, was of interest to the Swiss surgeon, Jacques Louis Reverdin (1842–1929). Reverdin experimented with a patient who had an open wound on his arm by taking a small piece of tissue from the healthy arm, which he embed in the granulation tissue of the healing arm. The small pieces attached themselves and the arm healed. This seeding of granulation tissue with normal tissue from another part of the body was known as a "pinch graft." In 1871, Stephen Chalker Bartlett performed the first skin graft on a woman whose hair had been caught in a revolving shaft, removing her entire scalp.

In order for grafting to make more progress, the advent of anesthesia would need to come into play because grafts, unlike flaps, took longer to accomplish and required more tissue to be transferred.

Z-plasties and New Techniques

Meanwhile, in Berlin, W. Hanff (1870) worked with the problem of revascularization, using frogs as his experimental model to study graft blood supply. Von Langenbeck (1810–1887) worked with transposition flaps from under the mandible. The flaps were quite successful but they left no tissue at the donor site, which often became infected. A recurring problem with donor sites was that after tissue was removed and taken for a different part of the body, another graft was required for the donor site.

Redundant eyelid skin surgery was of interest to Louis de Wecker (1832–1883) and Edmond Landolt (1845–1926) in Paris, who created a pedicle flap from the upper eyelid to use in a reconstruction of the lower eyelid. In Philadelphia, the dean of the medical school, William Edmonds Horner, had been passionately involved in one of the first pathology museums in the United States. Horner, a full professor of anatomy and editor of *Wistar's System of Anatomy,* collected samples of abnormal tissues for his collection and wrote a treatise on pathological anatomy as well as a dissection guide, with data gleaned from his studies of a variety of tissues. He named a tiny muscle of the eye the *tensor tarsi,* or *musculus hornerii*, and in 1837 worked on reconstructing eyelids and lips using a technique which cut the skin in a zig-zag fashion. This was the forerunner of the Z-plasty.

In 1854, in Montpellier, France, Michel Serre (1799–1849) and Charles Pierre Denonvilliers (1808–1872) worked on patients with ectropion, an unsightly condition where the lower eyelid is averted and the mucosal red surface is visible. This condition is characteristic of certain breeds of dogs, such as beagles, bassets, and bloodhounds. Correcting the condition requires precision and care because the eyelid is so narrow. Since the area is curved, precise cutting and suturing is a challenge for surgeons making this correction. To perform the excision, the surgeons used a series of small transposition flaps, instead of one large one. The surgery was so involved and complex that an entire subspecialty of plastic surgery developed, oculoplastic surgery.

One problem implicit with any plastic surgery is that the defect created by removing skin or tissue will form scar tissue, which, when healed, is not as elastic as normal skin. When the scar forms, shrinkage or contracture occurs. In order to change the way the surgical scars were resolved, certain doctors tried new flap designs. In Finland, Lars Törnroth created two triangular flaps and transposed them to prevent the contracting tension on the scar tissue. Then, in 1887, Paul Berger used this same double transposition flap for an ectropion. He published the results of his work in 1914. This technique came to be known as a *Z-plasty* and is the best choice for the correction of linear scars.

Flaps

Basically, all flaps work according to three principles: advancement, transposition, and rotation. An important caveat to remember and respect is that the length of the flap must not exceed the breadth, and a 50–50 ratio must be created in order to promote ideal healing with a minimum of scar tissue. When working with the face, the surgeon and patient's primary post-operative concerns are scarring and infection. One early 20th-century surgeon, Dr. Edmund Owen, specified how to avoid a scar when operating on a child's harelip. In his monograph (Owen 1904, 93), he details the procedures (i.e., "a thick wedge-shaped flap boldly tilted down so as to leave an angular space into which the opposite side of the lip . . . accurately dove-tailed").

Jacques Delpech continued this research but focused on other parts of the body, designing a rotation flap, a folded reconstruction for the lining of the lower lip. Dieffenbach (1792–1847), whose name was already known from his work with rhinoplasties, tendon repairs, and interest in body image and the psychological significance of scars, experimented with V-Y flaps on the lower lip. A V-Y flap was a type of advancement flap used to close an irregular-shaped wound.

Tubed Flaps

A number of early 20th-century dentists, physicians, and surgeons made strides in the techniques of plastic surgery, particularly the tubed flap. One benefit of the tubed flap was that the "suitcase" handle protected the raw tissue from local irritation. The Russian ophthalmologist Vladimir Petrovich Filatov (1874–1956) ("Editorial" 1975, 461) experimented with rabbits first and then successfully used the tubed flap technique on humans during the years of the Russian Revolution (circa 1916). This flap went from the clavicle (collar bone area) to the mastoid process (behind the ear). Filatov is best known for work with corneal grafts using cadaver donor tissue, and the keratoplasty which later became a popular, almost faddish, surgery. With this type of graft, the patient who previously wore eyeglasses no longer needed them to see objects that were far away. A keratoplasty is now performed with a laser and reshapes the cornea so that the correction allows for better distance vision.

In Germany, the dentist Hugo Ganzer (1879–1960) was considered a pioneer in facial reconstruction. He used a series of tubed pedicle flaps to repair the mouth and lower jaw of a patient. Using nasolabial flaps, he reconstructed noses, periorbital reconstructions, cleft palate repairs, and jaw reconstruction. Since he was trained in dentistry and not medicine, his contributions, although important, were not recognized or validated formally. Ganzer had studied medicine and biology, but chose to obtain a PhD instead of a medical degree; thus, he lacked the formal academic credential.

Victor Morax (1866–1935), a French ophthalmologist, originally trained in bacteriology. Although his primary work was in the treatment of eye infections, he became interested in plastic surgery, particularly the repair of

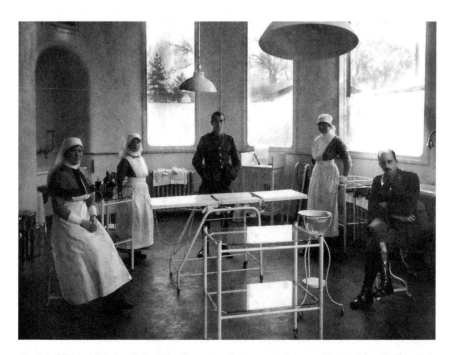

Harold Gillies (right) and staff in the cosmetic surgery theater, Queen Mary's Hospital, Kent, England, in 1917. Designed as the first plastic surgery center, doctors at the hospital performed more than 11,500 facial reconstruction procedures during World War I. (The Gillies Archives)

extensive defects that resulted from the removal of large tumors. He applied the tubed flap to an area on a patient's forehead that was too large to close after removing a nevus (large pigmented mole). Morax had performed a sophisticated flap procedure on a patient who needed lower eyelid repair on both sides. There, he used a flap from the patient's neck to fix the first lid. When it healed with adequate circulation, he detached it from the first lid and attached it to the second. The tubed pedicle flap later was used extensively by the surgeon Dr. Harold Gillies (1882–1960), who is also responsible for the successful launch of plastic surgery as specialty during wartime.

WARTIME INJURIES EVOLVE INTO THE SPECIALTY

The most significant plastic surgeon of the world war eras was the British surgeon Harold Delf Gillies, whose work in otolaryngology led to maxillofacial surgery and restoration of function. Gillies was daring, unconventional, and innovative. He combined artistry with medical expertise and devised a number of procedures to repair and restore severely damaged faces. The epithelial fold for constructing eyelids and lining the mouth, the pedicle flap, and transplants from one part of the skin to another were his most dramatic contributions. Because there were so many wounds requiring treatment, surgeons from all over the world were able to come to his centers to study and practice under his supervision. There was an ample supply of patients available in one location so the surgeons could do more than one surgery during their time with Gillies. His first book, *Plastic Surgery of the Face,* was published in 1920. Gillies credits Tommy Kilner, who worked closely with him and assisted with cutting grafts, for the success of the clinics at Dollis Hill and Treloar's hospitals. In 1931, Gillies teamed up with A. H. McIndoe and R. M. Mowlem, two other surgeons, who continued to fulfill the need for repairing and restoring war injuries. Because of the success and importance of the plastic surgery performed, when surgeons returned home after the war, they continued to use their new techniques and apply them to cosmetic and aesthetic surgery.

REFERENCES

"Editorial: Vladimir Petrovich Filatov." 1975. *British Journal of Ophthalmology* 59: 461.

Lyons, Albert S., and Joseph R. Petrucelli. 1987. *Medicine: An Illustrated History.* New York: Abrams.

Magner, Lois N. 1992. *A History of Medicine.* New York: Marcel Dekker.

Mütter, Thomas Dent. 1843. *Cases of Deformity from Burns, Successfully Treated by Plastic Operations.* Philadelphia: Merrihew and Thompson.

Owen, Edmund. 1904. *Cleft-Palate and Hare-Lip: The Earlier Operation on the Palate.* London: Baillière, Tindall and Cox.

CHAPTER 3

Challenges and Applications

The usual response to trauma is that tissue begins to heal. The first stage involves inflammation, a normal response, followed by necrosis, death of the injured cells and adjacent tissue. Finally, a specialized cell, known as a mast cell, is activated, which, in turn, stimulates the production of histamine. This process is referred to as an immune response. Histamine causes blood vessels to enlarge, which then increases blood flow to the damaged/healing area. Because the small blood vessels are more permeable, plasma and blood proteins flow into the area and cause swelling. However, once these proteins get into the injured area, a clot begins to form from the protein fibrin in the blood. At the same time, protective white blood cells called macrophages eat up the foreign proteins and prevent the injury from getting worse. The next phase in healing is the formation of scar tissue from the fibroblasts that moved into the area where cells died. The fibroblasts lay down a network of collagen fibers which, in time, will match the original tissue.

Every part of the body regenerates in a different way, and although the formation of scar tissue is necessary, it often leaves a traumatic result, particularly when a large amount of tissue has been destroyed. This formation of scar tissue is one of the biggest challenges for plastic surgeons.

Once the acute problem is solved and scar tissue is formed, the next challenge is to restore functionality. Did the patient undergo immobilization in order for the scar tissue to form? If so, then painful therapy is necessary to undo the effects of inactivity. Did the patient lose function because the scar tissue contracted in specific areas such as the head and neck? If so, useful therapies are found in the writings of Thomas Dent Mütter (1811–1859), who worked exclusively with these challenges for a majority of his medical career (Mütter 1843).

WORLD WAR I, OR THE GREAT WAR

Wartime injuries provided the greatest challenge for plastic surgeons simply because of the vast number of patients requiring immediate emergency treatment. Harold Delf Gillies, with a team of dentists, opened the first plastic surgery unit in Cambridge Hospital. This clinic became the model for others to learn repair techniques. However, it seemed that as soon as one facility opened, there was need for another. During the battle of the Somme, the team expected to treat 200 patients but 2,000 wounded individuals arrived. The biggest challenge was trying to encourage men to want to live, when they were unable to talk, taste, eat, sleep, or see. These poor souls would be wrapped in bandages, often unable to move. Damage from bullets and shrapnel caused horrific destruction to facial features. Tissue loss was difficult to compensate for when wounds could not be closed. To make matters worse, long delays after injury meant a greater opportunity for infection, requiring immediate treatment. Although emergency reconstruction lessened the chance of infection, the procedures often had to be undone and tissues realigned. A number of flaps were devised during this time period: local flaps such as the Bishop's Mitre flap, the Caterpillar flap, the Transposition flap, fat flaps and temporal muscle flaps were coordinated, often with the dental surgeons if areas of the face, mouth, jaws, or lips were involved.

One problem associated with dental surgery was that even if a bone graft could be performed because teeth were missing, without the *buccal sulcus* (hollow place in the cheek), dentures could not be constructed. Another problem was that although the dentists could work along with the anesthesiologists, often the problem of inadequate oxygen would require the stopping of surgery so that the patient could be ventilated. Sometimes the surgery was stopped and not finished because it was a choice between a successful surgery or a live patient. This was later solved by operating on a sitting, rather than a supine, patient.

Rhinoplasties, operations to restore damaged or missing noses, often employed flaps but frequently resulted in extreme tissue shrinkage. Through experience, surgeons learned that flaps had to be lined on the inside, as well, using a turn-over lining flap. An additional reinforcement with cartilage steadied and supported the nose when too much tissue had been destroyed.

One of the most important lessons learned was that although waiting too long gave infection the opportunity to invade, operating too soon had its disadvantages, as well. If a soldier's general health was poor and his level of hemoglobin was too low, it was not wise to operate. Since so many wartime injuries required multiple surgeries, and despite the pleas of the soldiers to complete everything as fast as possible, it was prudent to wait until adequate healing and scar formation occurred before going to the next stage.

SCARRING

In the late 19th century, the Austrian anatomist Carl Langer devised guidelines to minimize the amount of post-operative visible scar tissue. The incisions were made along a construct known as a skin tension line. He constructed a diagram of a human body showing all the places where skin was more amenable to being sutured. These lines became known as "Langer Lines." They provide the basis for a surgeon's decision regarding where to make the first incision in any operation or repair. Healing along Langer Lines results in a less-visible scar, or a propensity for the scar to diminish, eventually becoming invisible. Still, scars will occur and, sometimes, in trying to remove one scar, another will be created. One of the problems with removing a scar is that the edges will roll in slightly and cause a contracture. Another problem with scars involves the underlying tissue. If there is a difference in the two sides of the scar and one side lost more fat, muscle, cartilage, or bone, the excised scar will not heal evenly.

MUSCULAR ATROPHY

With any part of the body, inactivity and immobility will cause muscular atrophy. The complex problem of healing, even if infection can be controlled, is compounded when the body is kept without movement or exercise. On the one hand, delicate tissues must be kept inactive in order to heal. On the other hand, too much inactivity results in muscular atrophy. For example, the solution for some patients with nonhealing leg ulcers is to create cross-leg flaps that will not tear apart. Skin from the good leg is used as a donor site to be attached to the ulcerated area. The problem is that both legs must be immobilized until healing takes place. This is difficult for patients to tolerate. In the past, when the flaps healed, the leg muscles had atrophied and patients needed assistance to rebuild strength in order to walk. Early cross-leg flaps, prior to the age of antibiotics, were vulnerable to infection, a threat that loomed large in the face of any surgery.

HAROLD DELF GILLIES

The surgeon most frequently associated with the tubed flap is Harold Delf Gillies (1882–1960), a military surgeon from New Zealand. Although Filatov first used the technique in 1916, Gillies expanded its use to other areas of the body. Gillies's history as a plastic surgeon began in 1879, when he repaired burns on a sailor with extensive facial damage. Because of this successful restoration, patients who sustained facial injuries were often sent to him. In addition to physician referrals, patients who had heard of his reputation were referring themselves. Soon he assembled a team with Charles August Valadier, a dentist experienced in repairing jaw defects, and Kelsey Fry, another dentist. In 1917, they opened a hospital on the grounds of Frognal House, Sidcup, exclusively for servicemen who had sustained facial injuries during the war. Patients from all over the U.K. were transferred to Frognal House. It was the first wartime hospital of its kind and later became a teaching hospital for surgeons who wanted to join the team. It was called Queen's Hospital and was only intended to stay open for 10 years, but after the soldiers left it was maintained and renamed Queen Mary's Hospital. Henry Tonks (1862–1937), a British surgeon with a talent for painting, documented many of the procedures performed there with drawings and sketches of the surgical procedures. Tonks became an official war artist during World War I. Many hospitals developed art and photography departments to document and preserve the work their surgeons were performing so that the medical record would have artistic renderings along with the patients' medical histories (Gillies and Millard 1957).

Gillies was well aware of the confusing boundary between reconstructive and aesthetic surgery. In his view, reconstructive surgery was an attempt to return to normal, whereas aesthetic surgery was an attempt to surpass the normal. If a patient was a well-known entertainer whose livelihood depended on his or her appearance, and they requested plastic surgery to correct a blemish or imperfection, he saw no problem in complying with their request. There would be many more differences in opinions and attitudes regarding plastic surgery's boundaries. Gillies stressed that the psychological damage from an injured or flawed facial feature could result in an inferiority complex, a portmanteau term new to the medical specialty, psychiatry.

CONCOMITANT NEEDS OF THE PLASTIC SURGERY PATIENT

During this period, the specialty of psychiatry was growing as rapidly as plastic surgery. Alfred Adler (1890–1937), the Austrian psychotherapist, coined the term "inferiority complex" to describe the group of symptoms (i.e., low self esteem, feelings of inferiority, insecurity, inequality, and submissive behavior that contributed to form the complex). A colleague of Freud, Adler was a prominent visionary in the expansion of psychiatry. Freud's work with survivor guilt and its expression in conversion hysteria were important in treating soldiers who returned from wars.

Because of the massive limb trauma and resultant amputations, prostheses were created to compensate for losses that surgery could not repair. When World War I ended, the military surgeons returned home with skills that they could adapt to the traumas suffered by civilian populations. Thus, the specialty of plastic surgery developed on the battlefield continued to be honed on the domestic front. When the Society for Plastic and Reconstructive Surgery wrote their constitution, they wisely included the importance of social, economic, and psychological aspects of their specialty. In 1934, Gillies spoke to an American audience about the importance of psychological happiness. He addressed the growing concerns regarding cosmetic issues. Gillies did not feel that aesthetic surgery was frivolous, particularly if a person's livelihood depended on his or her appearance. Then the Second World War erupted and Gillies, now with two decades of experience, was able to use his skills on the soldiers injured in the latest battles. One of his techniques, the tubed flap, became a standard procedure and technique to use where circulation and infection were at risk. Because of his practice in the field and experiments on various parts of the body, tubed flaps could now be performed in any part of the body.

APPLICATIONS OF FLAPS

A multiplicity of types of flaps were invented and successfully employed during wartime. Civilian surgeons found such flaps useful in correcting genetic defects of the groin in male children. Flaps were devised so that the urethra could be reconstructed in the common genetic condition known as hypospadias, which is an abnormal opening on the underside of the penis. In this deformity, the opening for urine, instead of extending all the way to the tip of the glans, comes out on the underside of the urethral groove. Sir Astley Cooper and Benjamin Travers in England, Jacques Delpech in France, and Bernard Rudolph Conrad von Langenbeck in Germany worked with reconstructing urethras with hypospadias during the early to mid-nineteenth century.

The challenges described above were well on the way to being solved, but still required extensive time in the operating room and healing without any complications. Once a way was found to keep a patient comfortable during surgery and safe afterward, plastic surgery took another giant step forward. Anesthesia, essential to lengthy surgeries, could be administered with a greater margin of safety. Its story is an important chapter in the history of medicine.

REFERENCES

Gillies, Sir Harold, and D. Ralph Millard Jr. 1957. *The Principles and Art of Plastic Surgery.* Boston: Little, Brown and Company.

Mütter, Thomas Dent. 1843. *Cases of Deformity from Burns, Successfully Treated by Plastic Operations.* Philadelphia: Merrihew and Thompson.

CHAPTER 4

Anesthesia and Antisepsis

No matter how inventive and creative the advancement in plastic surgery, two challenges remained: pain and postoperative infection. Often, the thought of pain was enough to convince patients to forego surgery and accept death. Historically, there was evidence of the use of analgesics and anesthetics throughout the non-Western world. Opiates had been used in ancient India for the pain of nasal reconstruction; coca leaf was common in South Mesoamerica; *Datura stramonium* (jimson weed) was used in Asia and pre-Columbian America; and the poppy and cannabis were used in Egypt and Arabia. In Mesopotamia, Greece, and Rome, hyoscyamine, hemlock, lettuce-opium, and mandrake were known to produce somnolence or relieve pain (Lyons and Petrucelli 1987). All of these substances are toxic or poisonous when taken in large amounts; thus, Paracelsus's time-honored maxim, "The difference between a poison and a medicine is the dose." This succinctly summarizes the first rule of toxicology and the need for diligence when prescribing pain medications. The actual word *anesthesia* was coined in 1846 by Oliver Wendell Holmes, who combined the Greek words *an*, meaning "without," and *esthesia*, meaning "feeling."

Infections were puzzling to healers. The ancients had believed that the production of "laudable pus" was necessary for healing, when in actuality it was a sign of the body's response to a foreign bacterial agent. Yet, since no microscope had been built to view tiny creatures and the germ theory had not yet been proposed, the cause of infection was attributed to such disparate elements as an angry god seeking revenge or weather conditions.

Both contributions, anesthesia and antisepsis, which added in the advancement of plastic surgery and medicine in general, took place in the mid-19th century. Each was initially met with skepticism. Antisepsis was difficult to accept because microorganisms were invisible to the naked eye and without proof that such a phenomenon existed, hand washing or sterilization seemed to be only a ritual without scientific merit. Anesthesia, already proven to be a miraculous tool, challenged a certain religious mentality because it was thought that if God intended for people to experience pain, then it was immoral for a doctor to remove it. Each was eventually accepted as necessary and used concomitantly, allowing more time for surgeons to have a patient asleep or pain free with topical, local, open or closed general induction delivery methods systems.

EARLY PAIN CONTROL

Worldwide, the first anesthetics are not well documented in the medical literature. They have been described as coarse methods like a blow to the head severe enough to cause a concussion, drinking enough alcohol to become unconscious, or blood-letting until the patient became almost comatose. However, there is no real proof that any of these methods were ever used. Obviously, there were high risks of failure, permanent brain damage, or even death. Some early woodcuts of Johannes Scultetus (1595–1645) illustrated a woman undergoing a mastectomy, with heavily lidded eyes and lips near a straw. Perhaps this depicts her under the influence of some pain-numbing liquid. Prior to Scultetus's time, the *spongia soporifera* was used throughout Italy and Europe. An anesthetic sponge was prepared from opium, mandragora, hyoscyamine, and mulberry juice. These elements would be pulverized, immersed in liquid, and then soaked up by a sponge. The sponge was then dried. Just prior to surgery, the sponge would be dampened and placed in the patient's mouth. The patient would be instructed to inhale and the vapors of the drugs until they were gradually lulled to sleep.

GASEOUS ANESTHETICS

It wasn't until the 18th century that nitrous oxide inhalation was tried for medical purposes. Previous to the discovery of its medical significance, nitrous oxide was a party drug: it made people laugh. Partygoers under its influence could stub a toe or run into the corner of an end table and not feel any pain until the next day. This quality of un-feeling was recognized by a young English surgeon's assistant, who suggested that it could be used as an anesthetic. But, since he was viewed only as a trained but uneducated worker, his idea was ignored. In 1799 Sir Humphrey Davy published an article about the possibility of using nitrous oxide gas for surgical operations. One year later, William Allen, a physician at Guy's Hospital, is credited for demonstrating the use of nitrous oxide on a patient during surgery, but it was not until 1842 that Crawford Long removed a tumor from the neck of a patient who was sedated using nitrous oxide.

Ether was another drug first used recreationally and later tested during surgical procedures. Exactly who used it first and where is complicated enough to fill a book. Basically, physicians, chemists, and dentists share the "first implementer" occupational honor. England, New England, and Georgia all record events where inhalation anesthesia was successfully used. Robert Liston (1794–1847) in England; Crawford Long (1815–1878), a physician in Georgia; William Thomas Green Morton (1816–1868), a dentist in Massachusetts; Horace Wells (1815–1848), a dentist in Connecticut; and Charles T. Jackson (1805–1880), a Massachusetts physician, each contributed to the glory and fame associated with this miraculous adjunct to medicine.

Chloroform, Ether, and Nitrous Oxide

The English obstetrician James Young Simpson (1811–1870) had been searching for a drug to use on women during childbirth (Lyons and Petrucelli 1987, 518). Interestingly, chloroform's discovery (trichloromethane) was shared by three independent individuals: Samuel Guthrie (1782–1848) in the United States; Eugene Soubeiran (1797–1859), a pharmacologist, in France; and Justus von Liebig (1803–1873) in Germany. Like ether and nitrous oxide, chloroform, too, was a party drug and Simpson inhaled the gas and found that the aroma of chloroform was more fragrant than that of ether or nitrous. For about 10 years, the three gases remained recreational drugs, with no acceptable medical use until Horace Wells experimented by using nitrous himself and allowing someone to pull one of his teeth. Morton and Wells then began to experiment with ether and when they felt secure enough that it really did work, contacted the Harvard physician John Warren, who demonstrated this newest boon to medicine on October 16, 1846. This anniversary is now referred to as "Ether Day" by medical historians and in medical history documents (Fenster 2001). The first documented use of ether in plastic surgery was performed by the Jonathan M. Warren, the son of John Warren, one of the founders of inhalation anesthesia. Simpson, now in Scotland, preferred chloroform instead of ether for his obstetric and gynecological patients because it took less time to induce. Ether was safer and less toxic, but chloroform remained the anesthetic of choice in the United Kingdom. Conversely, South America, France, Sweden, Portugal, Spain, and Cuba embraced ether as their anesthetic of choice. The German plastic surgeon Friedrich Dieffenbach (1795–1847) wrote, "The wonderful dream that pain has been taken away from us has become reality. Pain, the highest consciousness of our earthly existence, the most distinct sensation of the imperfection of our body, must bow before the power of the human mind, before the power of ether vapor" (530).

In 1881, the chemist August Freund discovered the gas cyclopropane. But cyclopropane wasn't used for anesthesia until 1929 when the chemist George Lucas and pharmacology professor Velyien Henderson began experimenting with the gas on cats, kittens, and rabbits. They found that the gas affected respiration first, then blood pressure. By gradually decreasing the dosage, they could safely bring the animal up from a deep sleep. Cyclopropane became a frequent inhalation anesthetic for humans, often used in conjunction with ether and halothane.

TOPICAL AND LOCAL ANESTHETICS

A topical anesthetic is one that is applied to the skin or mucous membrane without penetrating the tissue. Often, a topical is applied prior to the injection of a local anesthetic, which is delivered to a subcutaneous or intramuscular part of the body. These anesthetics allow the patient to remain awake but pain-free during surgery.

Cocaine

The first medicinal application of topical and local anesthetics was introduced by Karl Koller in 1884 when he applied cocaine to the conjunctiva during ophthalmic surgery. Cocaine gained its god-like reputation from the psychotherapist Sigmund Freud (1856–1939), who promoted its use as if it were a panacea. Cocaine produced mental stimulation, provided a treatment for depression, cured digestive disorders, and reversed the craving for those addicted to morphine. After Freud developed cancer of the jaw, he was able to assuage the pain by using cocaine. Because cocaine was absorbed by mucous membranes, it was extremely useful in nasal and dental surgery. It was applied with a cotton swab. Most topical anesthetics could be sprayed or injected into small areas, usually mucous membranes that would absorb the molecules, to allow for painless injections of local anesthetics, if warranted.

After the invention of the hypodermic needle in 1853, the doctor, nurse, or surgeon designee could inject cocaine or another local anesthetic under the skin. Both Alexander Wood (1817–1884) and Charles Pravaz (1791–1853) are credited with this technology. The advantage of injecting a local anesthetic during facial plastic surgery is that it leaves the operating field free from the clutter of a mask and tubes, both necessary to administer anesthesia by inhalation.

INJECTABLE GENERAL ANESTHETICS

The barbiturate group of sedatives was developed in the early 1920s and Nembutal was introduced in 1930. Another class of drugs, prepared from curare, a plant used in South America to paralyze game during hunting, was added to the operation room armamentarium. Curariform drugs such as tubocurarine found its application in surgical procedures because it guaranteed that involuntary muscular movements would not occur while the patient was asleep and the doctor operating. However, in order for this to be successful, oxygen had to be administered during surgery in order to artificially inflate the lungs, because curare paralyzed all muscles, including the diaphragm. If the diaphragm did not expand and contract, the patient could not breathe. Injectible anesthesia, along with administration of oxygen, made lengthy and complicated surgeries possible. Later, hand washing, the use of gloves and drapes, and wound cleaning using an antibacterial substance (although the word antibacterial had not yet been coined), added to the increased rate of survival after surgery.

ANTISEPSIS

Infections had a propensity to develop after grafts. Since no accurate worldwide statistics regarding success were kept, one can only guess that the failure rate of surgeries due to infections was quite high. Since antisepsis by definition means "against infection," doctors first needed to learn what caused an infection before they could fight it. That history includes three scientists who explored the reasons that meat spoiled and milk soured, basically the causes of decay and putrefaction. Francesco Redi (1626–1697) had tried to disprove the theory called spontaneous generation, the belief that organisms arose spontaneously in substances. He demonstrated that maggots did not appear on meat as it spoiled unless an agent, such as a fly, laid eggs on its surface. If the meat was kept from the air and contact with flies, no maggots appeared. However, the human mentality, accustomed to traditional belief rather than independent observation, could not accept that truth. Lazzaro Spallanzani (1729–1799) demonstrated that boiled meat juices poured into a flask which was then sealed so that no air could contact the broth would not spoil. Later, Louis Pasteur (1822–1895), whose work on fermentation defined "a living form which originates from a germ," added to the growing knowledge regarding microorganisms (Garrison 1929). Closely related to the work of Pasteur was the bacterial work of Robert Koch (1843–1910), which led to the isolation of the anthrax bacillus, proving the sequence of how disease is spread by microorganisms and how one can isolate the causative agent, and how to introduce it into a new host.

Now that the agents for disease, sepsis, and infection were identified as enemies to the organism—a huge step in medical science—methods to abolish them was the next challenge. Joseph Lister (1827–1912), whose careful surgical amputations failed to yield a survival rate higher than

45 percent, had tried to keep his post surgical patients' wounds scrupu-lously clean. But despite his care, they continued to die, often demonstrat-ing laudable pus, a sign mistakenly believed to be beneficial to healing. Lister observed that when wounds healed without laudable pus, they healed by primary intention, where each part of the incision forms a ma-trix of tissue and grows together. More of his surgeries were successful and more patients lived beyond the post-surgical phase.

Antisepsis was barely accepted and sporadically practiced: sterile technique with masks, gloves, drapes, and clean instruments had yet to be standard practice. Despite the painstaking work of Ignaz Semmelweis (1818–1865), with his meticulous statistics about the direct relationship between sepsis and childbed fever, his figures were ignored. Doctors went directly from the morgue after performing autopsies to the delivery room and infected healthy women, who died soon after the procedure. He had found that simply washing hands in a solution that contained phenol after leaving the morgue and before examining women in labor would prevent infection. Unfortunately, his colleagues would not accept the information. He lectured on the importance of cleaning pus and blood off of hands that would touch multiple patients, but the concept of "germ" had yet to be discovered or recognized as the etiology for disease. Semmelweis knew there was a causative agent that was transmitted from decomposed bod-ies to healthy ones, but also that that "something" was neither seen nor understood.

It would be another 20 years before Joseph Lister (1827–1912) pub-lished his work on the treatment of wounds with carbolic acid (phenol), based on the principles of Pasteur's work with bacteria. Lister found that he could prevent the spread of necrosis by cleaning the site with a rag soaked in this chemical. He had experimented with treating abscesses, compound fractures, and gangrene with antisepsis and then hypothesized that if severe forms of wounds could heal using carbolic acid, so could in-cised wounds.

Neither infection nor tissue rejection were understood as reasons why some grafts failed. Elie Metchnikoff (1845–1916) studied phagocytosis, the immune system mechanism by which a cell can engulf, destroy, and digest an invading organism. But the complex workings of the immune system and the specific cells and organs that are responsible for preserv-ing health of the individual were not known until the latter part of the 20th century.

MORAL AND ETHICAL BOUNDARIES

Prior to the advent of anesthesia, plastic surgery on very young patients was limited. In the 17th century, young children were kept awake for long hours prior to an operation so that they would fall asleep from exhaustion, often aided by a glass of wine. In certain parts of Europe, a philosophical dilemma ensued. Did a surgeon have the right to correct a deformity that God had created? One solution to the question was that if the patient underwent a religious ritual such as Holy Communion, absolution was granted and the child could have surgery. In medicine, a rationale for disease often exists. Some people believe that illness, deformity, or pain is "God-given" and therefore a test or a cross one must bear. The amount of intervention that a physician can prescribe or perform has been questioned throughout the centuries. When anesthesia was first used to modify the pain of childbirth, some of the first societal outcries accused doctors of meddling with God's message that women should bring forth children in sorrow. This so-called moral issue continues to stimulate provocative discussions and debate among physicians, lawyers, religious specialists, and ethicists in other fields of medicine. Certain fundamentalist beliefs teach that the body should not be decorated or altered. In America, there were no controversies regarding cleft palate and cleft lip repair, although, later on, certain plastic surgery procedures were subject to ethical questions regarding informed consent and at what age a patient could make a decision. One of the early arguments that persuaded those originally opposed to anesthesia for moral reasons to accept it was that God had caused a deep sleep to overcome Adam when he removed the rib from his body to create Eve. However, once anesthesia was accepted as both moral and safe, plastic surgery on children and others could be more complex and of longer duration. The surgeon would not be competing against time and could, therefore, concentrate on the surgery rather than on the patient's pain. The final sutures to close surgical wounds required precision and time; thus, anesthesia was a boon to this crucial stage in the operation.

REFERENCES

Fenster, Julie M. 2001. *Ether Day.* New York: HarperCollins.
Lyons, Albert, and R. Joseph Petrucelli. 1987. *An Illustrated History of Medicine.* New York: Abrams.

CHAPTER 5

Wartime: The Mother of Invention

Humans are credited with having the largest brains in proportion to their bodies and the highest intelligence of all living creatures, yet they excel in finding ways to exterminate each other. From the earliest fossil evidence found in Africa to the most recent slaughters worldwide, ancient bones and modern corpses demonstrate the ways that people have invented to maim and kill. The noble-savage myth of the 19th-century philosopher Jean Jacques Rousseau is obviously an oxymoron. No group of people has ever existed without threat from an outside society or aggression from within in the form of the "other." Even the sacred book of the Judeo-Christian tradition, the Bible, tells stories of battles and wars, conflicts where people are smote with a sword or burned. Although the earliest technologies such as rocks, flint arrowheads, and knives could maim and kill, as societal conflicts evolved from tribal warfare to statehood armies, more complex weapons were invented. And as societies grew, so did the numbers of individuals injured in warfare.

The Chinese invention of gunpowder, a combination of charcoal, sulfur, and potassium nitrate, circa 1000 CE, provided both entertainment in the night skies and fierce destruction. Gunpowder by itself was impressive, but when it was loaded into metal holders, it provided the necessary ingredient for the first firearms, something capable of causing severe injury. The combination of gunpowder and metal pipes or tubes was adopted by the Arab and Asian worlds, each in unique ways, and by the 15th century, was well established as an ideal weapon.

The best surgeons could do for gunshot wounds was to clean and debride the flesh, hopefully to restore function, but doctors and barber surgeons did not understand too much about anatomy or physiology. Medicine was empirical, using techniques that appeared to work but not without what we now call an evidence base. Therefore, if a substance appeared to work, it continued to be used regardless of whether it contributed to healing or merely did not interfere with normal healing. Progress in surgery was slow because tradition was more important than innovation. It would take an usual doctor to change accepted dogma regarding wound treatment. Ambröise Paré (1510–1590) was such a doctor. In the world of Paré, cautery with a hot iron or boiling oil was the standard treatment for gunshot wounds. Serendipity in the form of an oil shortage reduced Paré's treatment choices, so he applied ointment and a bandage to the burn rather than allow it to go untreated. When he observed that healing accelerated at a faster pace using ointment and a bandage than with oil or cautery, he continued to use this new method. Paré's other inventions were the creation of prosthetic limbs and a method of terminating bleeding by tying off blood vessels. His changes and the quick acceptance illustrates how the increased number of injured people during wartime allows for more experimentation and innovation in medicine than in any other circumstance.

WARTIME ADVANCEMENTS

The wars of "civilized" nations have given surgeons the opportunity to use their new techniques to erase the disfigurements caused by an ever-growing armory of weapons. While World War I raged between Serbia, Austria, France, Germany, Russia, Belgium, and Great Britain, American physicians, dentists, and nurses from Harvard, Columbia, and Johns Hopkins traveled to France to study injuries and restore faces destroyed by the war industry. To restore only function to these severely damaged faces was not enough: people also wanted to look human. For severely scarred individuals, cosmetic surgery played a crucial role in the final stage of their healing. The balance between reconstructive and cosmetic surgery was evident in these patients. Since the face is the primary social venue for human communication and interaction, one needs to be presentable and acceptable for ongoing relationships. Attractive people are easily accepted and validated, whereas when one is disfigured, the comfort level of the beholder is often challenged. Ease of acceptance applies equally to how a person sounds and how easily they communicate.

World War I

The surgeon credited with advances in making plastic surgery a global specialty was Harold Delf Gillies, an ENT military surgeon from New Zealand who worked in Covent Gardens in London when World War I broke out. He went to France with the Red Cross in 1915 and there met the dentist who would become instrumental in the success of his repairs: Charles August

Valadier. Valadier invited Gillies to work with him after he convinced the British General Headquarters that they needed a jaw and plastic unit. Gillies's notoriety as a plastic surgeon began in 1916, when he repaired burns on a sailor with extensive damage to his face. Because of this successful restoration, patients who sustained facial injuries were often sent to him.

Because of massive limb trauma and the resultant amputations, prostheses were created to compensate for those losses that surgery could not repair. When World War I ended, the military surgeons returned home with skills that they could adapt to the traumas suffered by civilian populations. Thus, the surgery developed on the battlefield continued to be honed and preformed on the domestic front. It is estimated that because of these plastic surgery units during World War I, 15,000 reconstructive procedures were performed which established Plastic Surgery as a new specialty.

After their extensive work with war victims, plastic surgeons with military experience were now recognized as experts in reconstruction of facial trauma and grafting for burn damage. American surgeons trained in otolaryngology were increasingly frustrated by the competition and exclusivity of plastic surgeons who politically controlled access to hospital operating room privileges and professional memberships. Instead of challenging a no-win situation, they traveled to Europe, specifically to Berlin, to meet and study under Jacques Joseph (1885–1934). Joseph's face-lifting technique became standard practice.

Among the American travelers to Berlin was Samuel Foman (1889–1971), an anatomist, who had the desire to learn as much as possible about cosmetic plastic surgery. His quest was successful, and after organizing his knowledge into teachable segments, he began to hold courses for otolaryngologists in 1940 (Santoni-Rugiu and Sykes 2007).

World War II

When World War II erupted, Gillies, now with two decades of experience, was able to use his skills on those soldiers. In 1939, Rooksdown House, a converted mental hospital, was equipped with an operating room and wards. Orthopaedic surgeon James Cuthbert, dental surgeon Martin Rushton, anesthetist Pat Shackleton, and nurse Dorothy Whiteside comprised his initial staff. The United States had not yet entered the war when Gillies traveled to Chicago, then South America, to lecture on his work. When he returned, teams were trained and then dispatched all over the world: two teams went to Cairo and Alexandria in Egypt; one to India to care for soldiers from Burma; another to North Africa (Gillies and Millard 1957). Since there was no Internet in those days, communication by mail went back and forth with questions about wounds and advice on grafting. The first brochure was printed and distributed with instructions on burns and closure of certain types of wounds so that soldiers could continue to fight despite their injuries. After D-Day (June 6, 1944), an epidemic of infections broke out in one hospital, ruining many of the grafts and flaps. A team of pathologists was called in to identify the germ (A-12 streptococcus), but it took months before they could eradicate it. The tubed flap became a standard technique where circulation and infection were at risk and special rooms were set aside for these patients. No floor sweeping was allowed when dressings were being applied and hospital staff did the best they could to maintain a hygienic environment. This was before they could obtain penicillin, when only sulfa was available.

AFTER THE WORLD WARS

During World War I, the plastic surgery units treated gunshot wounds and injuries from shrapnel. The burn cases were sent to general hospitals and, unfortunately, there was not too much that could be done for them. Grafting was still in its early stages. As the new warfare technologies of World War II created new types of injuries, new methods of skin grafts, pressure dressings, tube pedicle, and reconstruction with multiple pedicles were developed. When penicillin became available, many wounds healed faster when treated with powdered antibiotic and left to dry in fresh air instead of under a bandage. A dressing trapped moisture, the ideal place for bacteria to multiply. So, even though a dressing protected the skin from additional trauma, it also created a dark wet environment, perfect for harmful microorganisms to be able to reproduce.

Lip surgery with double-sided flaps, ear surgery, and tube pedicles using mucous membrane, fan flaps, full thickness flaps, and a variety of flaps were developed by the time of the Korean War. The wounds produced in this war destroyed mucous membrane and facial bones more than skin because of the weapons used. These defects presented more challenges to the plastic surgeon. Technology in the form of external appliances such as fixators was invented to hold devices in place while tissues healed. These were bars, splints, joints, and frames to support parts of the face. Dental surgeons created wires to stabilize broken jaws so that the teeth could be aligned while the jaw healed. Again, the pattern of bringing home wartime techniques to use in civilian populations was repeated.

REFERENCES

Gillies, Harold, and D. Ralph Millard. 1957. *The Principles and Art of Plastic Surgery.* Boston: Little, Brown and Company.

Santoni-Rugiu, Paolo, and Phillip Sykes. 2007. *A History of Plastic Surgery.* New York: Springer Verlag.

CHAPTER 6

Paradigm Changes in Reconstruction and Aesthetics

Plastic surgery encompasses a variety of procedures, some to restore function and others to enhance appearance. A third category could be considered, because many reconstructive procedures now result in improved appearance (even though initially the surgery was not intended to affect appearance). Certainly any defect, whether sustained in a traumatic event or occurring at birth, will likely promote some type of psychological damage in the individual. Long before surgeries were perfected, individuals remained healed but severely mutilated, particularly after a war where damage was extensive and scar tissue remained. Before implants, only a mask or prosthesis could cover the missing tissue. No one could argue that these individuals did not deserve some type of restoration to normalcy.

Obviously, severe scarring and disfigurement is not normal in American culture. However, certain African cultures incise decorative cuts on their members' faces as a cultural tradition, and those scars are regarded as admirable and beautiful by the indigenous people. At one time, in Germany, the mark of an upper-class and elite individual was a dueling scar or fencing scar known as renommierschmiss. This late 19th-century custom was viewed as prestigious because it signified power, bravery, and strength. At one time, the ideal body build in Western cultures was muscular and heavy, at another tall and slim. In America, the epitome of beauty changes with each generation, and not only the WASP (White Anglo-Saxon Protestant) majority. The radical "black is beautiful" paradigm no longer dominates African American culture. The wild Afro hair style is rarely seen and Dashikis are worn more often by recent immigrants than rebellious counter-culture advocates. Interestingly, many first-generation immigrants do not seek to obliterate their differences. College campuses host a variety of students from other cultures who feel free to wear their traditional garb or modify it in interesting ways. At one university in Florida, girls wearing headscarves that completely cover their hair, dress like other young people wearing tight jeans, summery tops, and high heels.

Unlike college campuses, where diversity is the norm, local communities tend to be more homogenous with respect to socioeconomic status. In a community where the majority of individuals is affluent and trendy, there will be more requests for surgery to exaggerate certain features such as plumped-up lips, breasts, and facelifts; in a community composed of working-class individuals, plastic surgery, if financially feasible, will be used to correct rather than enhance. Television has glossed over the relevant facts regarding plastic surgery and presents the populace with what is possible in Hollywood, California, as if it were without side effects, risk factors, or the fact that standards change. The history of reconstruction and its relationship to aesthetics helps the potential patient to understand that despite TV and glamorous images, plastic surgery is medicine, not fashion, and it is important to know the difference.

RECONSTRUCTION AND AESTHETICS

In the 18th century, the German surgeon Carl von Gräefe (1787–1840) published *Rhinoplastik.* He practiced rhinoplasty, like Gasparo Tagliacozzi's (1546–1599) and other Italian predecessors, by using a forearm graft, but unlike the 16th-century pioneers, he freed it instead of allowing it to remain attached. Cautious to an extreme, von Gräefe spread out his surgeries with three to four months in between to assure himself that the tissue sectioned the graft would be viable. He referred to his technique as *von Graefe's modification of the Italian method.*

Plastic surgery performed for purely cosmetic or esthetic reasons did not develop until later in the 19th century. In Germany, Jacques Joseph (1865–1934), also known as Jakob Lewin Joseph, completed his training assisting Professor Doctor Julius Wolff in Berlin. During that time, a mother approached him about her son, who had large, protruding ears. The boy was so humiliated and teased that he would no longer attend school. The woman begged Joseph to fix her son's ears, although at the time, Joseph could find no previous documentation of such a procedure. He operated on the boy and reported it to the Berlin Medical Society for publication— as one usually did when performing a unique or new surgery—assuming that his technique would be praised and accepted. But instead, Wolff fired him, ostensibly because he had operated outside of the expected and ordinary parameters of surgery. Perhaps Wolff was merely envious that he had not thought of plastic surgery's application to cosmetic rather than medical goals. In any event, this was a purely cosmetic operation with no functional change other than a decidedly positive psychological outcome for the young patient.

RACIAL AND GENDER ISSUES

John Orlando Roe (1848–1959) of Rochester, New York, worked with rhinophymas, a common condition where the nose becomes red, bulbous, and deformed, often associated with chronic alcoholism. His patients were Irish immigrants to the United States who felt that their status as citizens was inferior because of their noses. The typical "Irish" nose was a snub or pug nose and did not look like the typical "American" nose, which was longer and straighter. Roe classified noses into five types: Roman, Greek, Jewish, Snub/Pug, and Celestial. The snub or pug nose (he felt) indicated weakness and lack of development, a subject of melancholy interest and, according to some, proof of the degeneracy of the human race. This was a time in history where anthropomorphics and craniometry, the "science" of measuring the skull, played an important part in biology and criminology. Science had declared that certain facial and bodily features indicated personality types and propensity for crime. Darwin's concept of biological evolution was misused more than it was understood and social Darwinism, an inaccurate and unscientific way of looking at people, emerged. Anthropologists measured skulls and created categories of classification, indices that were only for identification purposes. Brain and skull size were supposed to be important indicators of intelligence, until the scientists discovered that one of their own had a very small brain. Women were allegedly less intelligent than men until the brain size-to-body size ratio was submitted as evidence and, in fact, according to the resultant hypothesis, women were more intelligent than men. Researchers, such as Paul Broca, attached meaning to normal human variability. For example, the facial angle defined how much the face, jaws, and cranial index represented a mathematical ratio of the width to the length of the skull. A dolichocephalic skull (a long skull from front to back, with an index of .75 or less) was long from front to back; a brachycephalic skull had an index of .8 or more. It was thought that those who possessed long skulls were more intelligent than those with short skulls, until racist researchers found that many African skulls, which were supposed to be more primitive and closer to apes, were dolichocephalic (Gould 1981). Then the paradigm changed, so that it was the short, wide Germanic skull that was the preferred skull shape. The pug noses that were maligned among the Irish in the 19th century became the desired noses of second-generation Jewish immigrants (Gilman 1999). Each wave of newcomers to American had distinctive facial characteristics, and many desired to eradicate those differences by virtue of cosmetic plastic surgery.

"Passing"—in what was then the dominant social group—as a WASP gave plastic surgery the impetus to expand its horizons beyond rhinoplasty. Historically, for many people, it was important to disguise their social class and ethnicity because there was so much prejudice in America against immigrants with certain physical features such as a pug nose, a large nose, an epicanthic eyefold, or large buttocks.

FACIAL PLASTIC SURGERY

Surgery for the exclusive purpose of improving appearance started in the 19th century, with the practice of removing what was considered a stigma of ethnicity or disease. Syphilis often caused a condition known as saddle nose, where the bridge of the nose is destroyed and the nose appears typically caved in. Early rhinoplasties were performed to repair noses that had been amputated as a punishment (see Chapter 2). Operations to repair scar tissue from burns or to correct cleft palates or harelips were certainly medically necessary. Later surgeries were performed to mask ethnic identity among those groups who felt that their appearance was a detriment to comfortable assimilation in a new country. All of these operations for the repentant criminal, the immigrant who does not conform to the status quo of the time period, and the deformed at birth or mutilated by accident attempted to improve appearance by restoring normality or to change unwanted features to be as acceptable as possible. Although physicians had written tomes on improving the effects of aging as early as the 16th century, without antibiotics and anesthesia, the extent of available surgeries to eradicate those changes was limited. Promoting the fountain of youth through plastic surgery was to become one of the most challenging and controversial aspects of medicine. At what point did the standards of plastic surgery change from necessary to elective? And how did standards of beauty or acceptability play into those standards?

One of the first surgeons to actively promote cosmetic surgery was Charles Conrad Miller (1880–1950), from Chicago. He had taken some courses in medicine at the Hospital College of Medicine in Louisville, Kentucky, and was awarded a third-year scholarship for excellence in his school work. His education consisted of four years, although each year's session only lasted six months. This minimal education was normal for a doctor in the days before medicine became a standardized profession with ethical guidelines (Flexner 1910). Miller obtained an M.D. and set up an office, where he instructed country doctors on how to set up an operating room. He was something of a maverick, called both the father of modern cosmetic surgery and a quack. His first surgeries in 1907 were to remove crow's feet (i.e., the removal of nasolabial folds), and correction of excessively thick everted or inverted lips. He performed a variety of procedures on what he called *featural imperfections.* These imperfections included ears that were too prominent, noses that had dorsal humps, dimples, eyebrows, and tattoo removal. Charles Miller was a prolific writer and published more than 41 articles about the plastic procedures he performed. He published his own journal, *Medicine and Health,* which, conveniently, included coupons for his textbooks.

As the country entered the Great Depression in the 1930s, Miller's practice changed and he did less plastic and more general surgery. Perhaps it was a consequence of being sued by an unhappy patient, his involvement with patent medicines, or because of the changing economy. Whatever the reason, he was wise to recognize that many patients seek cosmetic surgery to compensate for insecurity in other aspects of their lives. He also was aware that despite the need for better education and certification, many operators were incompetent opportunists. In addition, he observed a third problem in the field, that being that cosmetic surgery appealed to vain people, "idle men and women who have nothing better to do than study themselves" When these people seek plastic surgery, they expect unrealistic transformations (Miller 1924).

In a prescient insight, Miller wrote that America worshipped youth and, because of that, certain women whose professions depended on their looks would be in need of plastic surgery. In advice to other potential surgeons, he wrote that no matter how beautiful a middle-aged woman was, it would be impossible to rid her of all signs of maturity without some scarring. In addition, they would seek more surgery as they aged but eventually it would be harder to disguise the ravages of time and it would become equally difficult to hide the scars from surgeries. Miller's contributions to the development of American plastic surgery attest to his holistic attitude, not only to the techniques involved in cutting and sewing, but also to the emotional needs of the patient and the limitations of plastic surgery.

On the other side of the Atlantic, in Germany, Eugene von Hollander (1867–1932) is considered a pioneer in facelifts, commonly referred to as a rhytidoplasty. In a facelift, wrinkles, furrows, jowls, double chins, and baggy eyelids are removed. Hollander perfected the surgery by identifying narrow strips of skin along the hairline that could be removed and the edges sutured together. This "lifted" the skin on the face toward the scalp, causing a tighter appearance and eliminating wrinkles. He did not publish this aspect of his work until the year he died. Most of his published work documented reduction mammaplasties, a much-desired operation, popular before the paradigm of beauty shifted and breasts were enlarged rather than made smaller.

Erich Lexer (1867–1937) made s-shaped excisions in the temporal region and elliptical incisions along the forehead and hairline. Instead of suturing the pieces in place, he stretched the skin and anchored it behind the ear (Santoni-Rugiu and Sykes 2007). Perhaps these surgeons could have been more prominent had they published and promoted their work earlier, but they chose not to, out of fear of criticism from their peers.

REFERENCES

Flexner, Abraham. 1910. *Medical Education in the United States and Canada.* New York: The Carnegie Foundation.

Gilman, Sander. 1999. *Making the Body Beautiful: A Cultural History of Aesthetic Surgery.* Princeton, NJ: Princeton University Press.

Gould, Stephen Jay. 1981. *The Mismeasure of Man.* New York: W.W. Norton and Company.

Miller, Charles C. 1924. *Cosmetic Surgery: The Correction of Featural Imperfections.* Philadelphia: F.A. Davis.

Santoni-Rugiu, Paolo, and Phillip Sykes. 2007. *A History of Plastic Surgery.* New York: Springer Verlag.

CHAPTER 7

Corrective versus Cosmetic Surgery

Post–World War II society was ambivalent regarding the necessity of an expensive operation for something that had no urgent or traditional medical need. Doctors had seen the physical trauma and devastation of war repaired, but not necessarily healed, with plastic surgery. Antibiotics, anesthesia, and new technologies incorporated into the practice of medicine had changed its image and power. No longer exclusively a curative or emergency service, medicine's domain expanded, but at the same time returned to its original realm, that of a healing art. An additional dimension was that in order to secure that "art" to improve one's appearance, one required a lifestyle that could afford the price of surgery and the privacy to remain rested and away from the day-to-day stresses of life during the healing process. Not too many people had both the leisure time and the money to pay for such luxuries.

PARAFFIN, GUTTA PERCHA, AND FAT TRANSPLANTS

Although paraffin injections had been tried by Dr. Robert Gersuny in Vienna in the 1890s, they had been unsuccessful, because of the inflammation and irritation the injections caused in surrounding tissue. Paraffin injections were used to close defects in subcutaneous tissues. Charles Conrad Miller, referred to above, experimented with introducing a series of foreign substances for rebuilding purposes, and found that all caused painful or infectious reactions. In addition to infection, postoperative problems included migration or necrosis of the fat, which often left lumps or bumps, and absorption of the transplanted substance, which resulted in no change at all. Others surgeons tried, as well. In 1893, Gustav Albert Neuber (1850–1932) built up the tissue under the eye by implanting detached segments of fat; in 1896, Vincent Czerny (1842–1916) transplanted a lipoma (a benign tumor) to a breast; in 1909, H. Verderame reported that he used autologous fat transplants in ocular surgery. One consistent conclusion was fat transplants, in time, shrank and became absorbed, so a larger amount of fat had to be transplanted to compensate for the loss.

POST–WORLD WAR II

The entire social structure of the United States changed when World War II ended. Women, who before the war had originally been perceived as too weak to operate machinery or motor vehicles, were actually found to be excellent workers and took the place of those men who had to fight overseas. But now after proving they could perform tasks traditionally classified as for men only, they were forced to give up those jobs and return from military work to the home, once again relegated to their former "unskilled" roles as housewives and mothers. Men, returning from war, had to find work and took over the positions previously occupied by women. Many of those men suffered from emotional and physical trauma. Their faces, ears, noses, limbs, and extremities had been the beneficiaries of reconstructive surgery during the war and the results were impressive. Prostheses and physical therapy helped the amputees relearn many of the activities of daily living, and facial plastic surgery restored their outward appearance. Surgeons themselves debated whether a corrective rhinoplasty could be divorced from a reconstructive rhinoplasty, "corrective" being the ambiguous term. But the knowledge that a rhinoplasty was possible spread from the few to the many and the demand for plastic surgery continued to increase.

In 1923, the actress Fanny Brice had consulted a surgeon for a "nose job." Allegedly, she was interested in erasing her Semitic look to ensure acceptance by movie makers for future roles; this was at a time when prejudice against Jews was culturally prevalent in the United States. Brice denied the accusations that she was attempting to hide her Jewishness and blend in with the majority. In fact, she stressed that her nose, in any "language," was not attractive and she only wanted to look prettier. The question remains what constitutes "pretty"? Does pretty mean not looking like a member of an ethnic group? Statistics favor a trend that was expressed during the 20 years that followed the first waves of immigration from Eastern Europe. First- and second-generation Jews comprised more than half of those who sought rhinoplasty surgery. Then, in the 1940s, rhinoplasties in the United States increased again among Jewish people, perhaps because of the global fear generated by the Nazi holocaust and "racial purity" in Europe. In the 1950s, the typical rite of passage for a female teenager, in addition to a Bat Mitzvah, was a rhinoplasty. By the

mid-1960s, the upturned nose, which had suffered previous negative connotations for the waves of Irish immigration, was now the status symbol
of the upper-middle class Jewish teenagers living in New York City. Only
Barbara Streisand, a singer whose nose seemed to attract the attention of
every American magazine, dared to keep her Jewish nose unbobbed.

The target of remodeling and remaking the body moved downward
from the nose to the chin, breasts, hips, thighs, and calves. Magazines for
young women promoted plastic surgery as much as they did diet, clothing,
and relationship advice. Helen Gurley Brown, the editor of *Cosmopolitan*
and author *Sex and the Single Girl* and numerous advice books for women,
advised every female to have a facelift at age 40 before severe changes
occur, and regularly from that time on (Brown 1962).

BREASTS

Breasts have an interesting history in American culture. Breasts are
icons of primitive cultures, femininity, eroticism, maternity, power, and
sexual liberation. As signifiers of femaleness, their existence is compromised when cancer invades mammary tissue. Even if the woman has passed
the age of reproductive potential, the breast retains a powerful erotic con-
notation. So the ideal breast size and shape has always been the subject
of intense social focus. For many years, reduction mammoplasty was performed on women whose breasts were pendulous and large. At the t urn
of the 20th century, in certain countries, the perfect breast was regarded as
smallish rather than large, rounded rather than pendulous (Gilman 1991,
219). In Germany, a small firm breast was desirable because it connoted
youthfulness and athletic ability, as opposed to a breast that hung loosely,
associated with primitive societies. That particular viewpoint flew in the
face of the perky, self-supporting breast commonly displayed in *National
Geographic* magazines as native, unblemished, primal, youthful, and desirable. A generation of boys maturing in the 1950s found the breasts of
these women in exotic cultures certainly not unattractive or floppy.

Breast reduction had other purposes. Pendulous or excessively large
breasts were associated with obesity and lack of self-control. Hypertro-
phied breasts, in women of normal weight, in addition to being unattractive (to certain people) were heavy, caused backaches, and interfered with
sports activities. In order to compensate for the discomfort, a woman's
posture was compromised, and her appearance was burdened and dull.

Medical issues of graver importance, such as tumors or breast cancer,
required total or partial mastectomies. The female patient, faced with a life-
threatening malignancy, had to make a choice, which typically included a
total mastectomy. This often included removal of axillary lymph glands,
which resulted in edema and arm swelling because lymph could no longer

drain. Post-mastectomy, breast reconstructive surgery gave women a choice to look "normal," although some of the first implants obscured mammogram imaging and the "reconstructed" breast often did not match the intact remaining breast. Some surgeons advocated removing the healthy breast in addition to the cancerous one so that reconstruction could be performed to make both breasts identical. Surgeries to correct a complete mastectomy were more complex, requiring the construction of a new nipple and areola.

Plastic surgery was an accepted solution for those who suffered through procedures where large amounts of diseased tissue had to be removed. The radical mastectomy, a devastating surgical ordeal was often performed simultaneously with breast reconstructions using implants. Previously, women who survived radical mastectomy wore prostheses. These often slipped out, particularly in the water when put under a bathing suit top.

When total mastectomy was not necessary, a partial mastectomy was performed which spared the breast and the patient's self image. Reconstructions post-partial mastectomy involved taking tissue and fat from other parts of the body. Dermal-fat-fascia transplants are often used to reconstruct a breast, employing flaps to cover the surgical defect.

During the 1950s, the ideal female body type was obsessively modeled after Marilyn Monroe, Anita Ekberg, Gina Lollobrigida, and Jayne Mansfield—all large-breasted women. Monroe's blonde hair and small nose added to her appeal. Her all-American image adorned the cover and centerfold of the first issue of *Playboy* magazine in 1953, whose editor labeled her the sweetheart of the month. Her naked body, smile, and inviting facial expression served as the epitome in female beauty for many men. Even after the ideal female image changed to a small-breasted, slim-hipped female in the 1960s, the popular culture artist Andy Warhol memorialized Monroe in 1962 with a poster of airbrushed images in many colors.

Symbolically, it was time for women to wear the mantle of female domestic nurturers, not wartime factory workers. In these postwar years, the breast symbolized the reproductive virtue of a wifely woman—bearing and raising children. Yet the erotic breast, since it was forbidden, was obsessively desired and fetishized. Women wore push-up bras or padded bras. The bra manufacturer Maidenform advertised a variety of styles with such copy as, "I dreamed I was wanted in my Maidenform . . . I dreamed I went to a masquerade in my Maidenform . . . I dreamed I was queen of the westerns in my Maidenform . . . I dreamed I took the bull by the horns in my Maidenform." The bra supported and pushed up women's breasts so they appeared to be at a 90-degree angle from the floor and exaggerated the shape at the end of the nipples to appear pointed. It is not surprising that plastic surgeons were soon barraged with requests for mammary enlargement rather than reduction. Many such requests were anatomically unrealistic.

As is often the case with seemingly normal phenomena, breast size became "medicalized" and small breasts were called "hypo- or micromastia." Certain doctors, convinced of the potential market for a medical solution to this "problem," experimented with devices that could be implanted under the breast. One synthetic foam rubber (polyurethane) substance called "Surgifoam" was an early implant used for breast augmentation. The doctor who promoted it was neither a plastic surgeon nor a dermatologist nor a member of any boards or medical societies. The substance, known as Ivalon, was allegedly better than fat grafts, yet caused hardening and the formation of infiltration where breast tissue grew into the sponge pores. In some patients, the sponges shrank. Other materials, for example, Polistan, Etheron, and Hydron, were tried but none were without side effects. Some doctors had used liquid silicone injections but, although initially better than paraffin, the silicone tended to migrate.

Breast Implants

A new technology was needed. Paraffin, silicon injections, and the array of sponges had shown signs of failure as well as a litany of problems: migration, infiltration, masking of cancerous growths, infection, hematoma, and capsular contraction. In 1962, Frank Gerow, a surgical resident, observed an IV bag filled with saline and, thinking "out of the box," decided the form might be used as a breast implant. Together with Thomas Cronin, the staff surgeon, and Dow Corning, he worked on a flexible plastic bag that contained saline that could be inserted under the breast as an implant. The bag ultimately broke, but after experimenting with other substances as fill, they found that silicone gel was strong enough to withstand the pressure from chest tissues during breathing. To prevent migration of the implant, they used a piece of Dacron material as a patch that attached the prosthesis to the chest wall. The prosthesis was successful but the Dacron patch caused an inflammatory reaction. As they modified the implant design, they were finally able to do away with the patch. But there were still problems with capsule formation, a hard fibrotic mass that developed around the prosthesis much the same way an oyster forms a pearl from tissue irritation. In the 1970s, Franklin Ashley invented a silicone-gel implant covered with polyurethane foam that overcame the problem of encapsulation (Ashley 1970).

By the 1990s, almost 2 million breast implant surgeries had been performed. Outpatient surgery clinics opened so that the surgery could be done one day and the patient returned home the day after. The ramifications of this voluminous number of procedures will be addressed in the next chapter.

Regarding Personality

As the popularity and visibility of breast augmentation increased, so, too, did reports of improvements in mental health and happiness. So great was the emphasis on breast size that women were beginning to focus on their inferiority or psychological distress and project it onto their bodies. The extreme expression of this attitude is called body dysmorphic disorder (BDD) and it is a serious psychiatric problem. BDD is discussed in more detail in the second section of this book. Another negative consequence of the flurry of breast augmentation popularity involved issues surrounding safety and efficacy of silicone injections and sponge implants. Although some doctors stressed the importance of breasts in psychological satisfaction, others recognized that, in many cases, counseling would be just as effective. In those early days, few surgeons could predict how important a psychiatric screening would become for potential patients. It would protect both the patient and the doctor, because as the demand for plastic surgery increased, so did the number of lawsuits. Eventually, prudent plastic surgeons required that any patient desiring surgery would undergo an extensive interview and questionnaire to determine exactly what their expectations were.

Tissue Expanders

Massive tissue removal and breast replacement with implants were problematical, because once a tumor-laden breast was removed, there was a tissue deficit or defect. Often, if radiation had been used as an adjunctive treatment, the remaining skin would be difficult to use and not appropriate for a traditional graft because radiated tissue did not heal as rapidly as did untreated skin. Another problem was that if the cancerous breast had been extremely large, then there was not enough skin to cover the surgical site. To address these challenges, Hilton Becker in Boca Raton, Florida, started to experiment with a technique known as tissue expansion. Tissue expanders had been patented starting in the early 1980s, the first by Eldon Fritsch in 1984. He devised an expander that would convert to a breast implant after the healing tissues were modified to fit over the prosthesis. Previous expanders had required two steps: placement and removal. Typically, the expander is placed after the first surgery. Once the skin has expanded to efficiently cover the implant, a second surgery is performed to replace the expander with an implant. In Becker's technique, only one operation—a single-stage reconstruction—was necessary.

Some breast cancer patients choose to have the healthy breast removed along with the cancerous breast, to prevent any possibility of remission. With a total mastectomy, both the nipple and the breast are removed. For a subcutaneous mastectomy, the breast tissue is removed and the nipple remains. Finally, in an areolar-sparing mastectomy, the nipple is removed but the areolar tissue is converted to a nipple, with the surrounding tissue tattooed so that it looks like an areola. Because all or most of the skin and muscle are retained following a prophylactic mastectomy, the muscle is strengthened with an acellular dermal graft. While a flap can be used to replace the volume of the breast, the implant developed by Dr. Becker (the Mentor Becker 50/50) has been used to reconstruct the breast following prophylactic mastectomy.

TUMMY TUCKS (ABDOMINOPLASTIES)

Women whose pregnancies left them with stretched skin and flabby abdomens wanted to look "normal" again, so the need for "tummy tucks" developed. In the 1940s, the surgery was referred to as reconstruction of body contours due to grotesque deformities caused by hyperadiposity. Women who lost weight as a result of dieting recognized that they, too, could benefit from tighter skin if they underwent the surgery. Desire for these operations increased as more women, concerned about their weight, experimented with extreme diets that promised huge weight loss in very little time. The result of rapid weight loss was a large amount of abdominal skin, referred to as an apron. For patients who had surgery for breast cancer and subsequent augmentation mammoplasty, the operation doubly improved their appearance, because when abdominal fat along with the skin was removed to replace breast tissue, the result was a flatter stomach.

LIPOSUCTION

Liposuction is a technique for removing subcutaneous fat with a tubular pointed device attached to a suction machine. Prior to liposuction, in the 1930s, Jacques Maliniak surgically removed fat from the neck and face. Later in the 1950s, A. D. Davis used curettes to scrape out fat after making an incision under the chin. It was not until 1972 that the new, automated technology of liposuction was introduced. Josef Schrudde in Cologne took a cannula ordinarily used for gynecological surgery and modified it so that he could attach it to a suction device and remove fat particles from the face. He called this technique *lipexeresis.* By the late 1970s, doctors were routinely performing liposuction (removal of fat with a blunt cannula). Y. G. Illouz in France created a mixture of saline, hyaluronidase, lidocaine, and epinephrine that, when injected, caused the fat to dissolve (lysis). In 1987, Jeffrey Klein invented the "tumescent technique" of superficial liposuction that was used on the head and neck and involved a solution of lidocaine, epinephrine, and bicarbonate of soda.

Soon, a plethora of applications for liposuction appeared. More than small amounts of fat could be removed by targeting hips, thighs, the abdomen, arms under the triceps muscle, and almost anywhere in the body where adipose tissue collected. An unplanned problem related to the procedure was redundant skin, which hung like elephant skin, loose and in folds. Luckily, there was a surgical procedure to correct that as well, but the patient had to be warned not to gain weight after the procedures were completed.

THE RISE OF AN OUTPATIENT PROCEDURE

In 1981, the ophthalmologist Alan Scott first used botulinum to correct *strabismus* (crossed eyes) and blepharospasm (uncontrollable blinking, twitching, or fluttering eyelids) in humans, after experimenting with the substance on primates. The treatment corrected the condition but only worked for only a few months. Patients were then required to return for more injections. The toxin works by blocking the neurotransmitter, acetylcholine, a substance in the body that transmits nerve impulses to muscles. When the nerve is blocked, the muscle or muscles become paralyzed—this effectively removes wrinkles from skin, if only temporarily.

By 1998, the cosmetic application of the botulinum toxin (Botox) for removal of facial lines had increased by 1,500 percent in the United States, making Botox the most popular cosmetic procedure in the United States. The procedure is so ubiquitous, ostensibly safe, and accepted as routine that spas have arranged with plastic surgeons and dermatologists to sponsor events that provide the treatment. And with that introduction of neurotoxin to skin, we find the first cosmetic medical procedure that can be done on the go.

MALE PLASTIC SURGERY

Women are not the only patients who choose to have plastic surgery. Breast reduction in men is not talked about as often as it is in women, but approximately 40–60 percent of men have breast overdevelopment, though sometimes only unilateral (one-sided). Causes are not all known but certain drugs and hormonal therapy for prostate cancer will cause womanlike breast growth in men. Men with prostate cancer who had undergone hormonal manipulation often suffered the side effect of gynecomastia— the swelling of the mammary glands. Liposuction is useful to remedy that fat accumulation ("Patient Brochure" 1994).

Society, in general, regards male breast reduction as corrective rather than cosmetic and, therefore, justified. But where does necessity end and vanity begin? That is a difficult question to answer. In the 1990s, "dress for success" was a requirement, particularly since younger workers were challenging the Baby Boomer generation. The term "corporate downsizing" added to the anxiety of this group of male employees in banking, the stock market—formerly stable careers. The business world demanded youth, or at least attractive representatives, particularly in sales. Plastic surgery was no longer the exclusive domain of females. In addition to hair implants and using dyes to mask gray, men started to inquire about and undergo facelifts, brow lifts, blepharoplasties, Botox, laser skin resurfacing, neck lifts, and liposuction. Compared to 1980, when 10 percent of plastic surgery patients were male, in 1998, that figure had more than doubled to 25 percent (Man and Faye 1998). The growing self-improvement trend that started with the Yuppies now added the need for plastic surgery to the armament of diet and exercise. Men now underwent surgery for silicone implants when pectoral and calf muscle did not bulk up by exercise alone.

Male cancers of the prostate and testicles were often treated with orchiectomies (removal of the testicles). In consonance with the desire to look normal, testicular implants were designed to be put in the scrotal sacs. It is understandable that restoration of a body part amputated because of a deadly disease is both frightening and depressing. Just as breast implants are important to the body image of a woman who has had cancerous growths removed, so are testicular implants to some men.

REFERENCES

Ashley, Franklin L. 1970. "A New Type of Breast Prosthesis." *Journal of Plastic and Reconstructive Surgery* 45 (5): 414–24.

Brown, Helen Gurley. 1962. *Sex and the Single Girl.* New York: Random House.

Gilman, Sander. 1991. *Jews's Body (The).* New York: Routledge.

Man, Daniel, and L. C. Faye. 1998. *The Art of Man: Faces of Plastic Surgery.* Boca Raton, FL: BeautyArt Press.

"Patient Brochure." 1994. American Society for Plastic and Reconstructive Surgery Gynecomastia.

CHAPTER 8

Organizations and Societies

When the first group of dentists and surgeons met to establish the first formal organization for plastic surgeons, the founders recognized that because head and neck anatomy is complex, plastic surgery was multi-disciplinary. In a very small space, all the sensory organs, teeth, and individual characteristics that make each human distinct from each other are contained. That first group changed names and requirements many times before 1999 when the current group, the American Society of Plastic Surgeons, was named.

Wars, immigration, and the growing specialization of the medical profession led to the formation of the first association responsible for regulating and promoting plastic surgery. In 1921, three surgeons met in Chicago to form the American Association of Oral Surgeons. An early caveat of the association required all members to have obtained both a medical and a dental degree. Among the elected 20 founding members, only two had single degrees: one was a dentist and the other a physician. A few years later, the dental degree requirement was rescinded and in 1937, the name of the organization was changed to the American Association of Oral and Plastic Surgeons. The name was changed again in 1942 to the American Association of Plastic Surgeons (AAPS). During the 1930s, there were few preceptorships possible, and only five hospitals allowed plastic surgery services (St. Louis, Baltimore, New York, Boston, and London). Vilray P. Blair from St. Louis was concerned that some of the plastic surgery being performed in the United States was unacceptable and that patients were "often at the mercy of unconscious neglect of misdirected enthusiasm." He proposed that plastic surgeons should have general surgical training before they specialized, and brought his proposal to the American Board of Surgery (Simons n.d.). Earlier, an organizing committee of five had met and 11 others joined them to gain visibility. The American Board of Plastic Surgery was formed to insure that surgeons were getting sufficient training and oversight, and to set up guidelines. Their founding mission was seven-fold:

1. To establish standards of fitness to practice the specialty.
2. To arrange and conduct tests (examinations) for determining qualifications of those who profess to specialize in plastic surgery. And to grant certificates to those who meet the established standards set by the American Board of Plastic Surgery.
3. To offer or name specific conditions requisite to the certification in individual cases.
4. To act as preceptors or advisors to prospective students of plastic surgery.
5. To gather and promulgate reliable information as to the quality and practicability of various existing opportunities for the study of this type of surgery and to encourage furtherance of such opportunities.
6. To make constructive suggestions that promise advancement of the science for the practice of this branch of surgery.
7. To establish and foster a working relationship between the American Board of Plastic Surgery and the various special surgery boards sanctioned by the American Medical Association (AMA) as well as by the American Board of Surgery.

The association was connected to training programs in university-based medical schools to further solidify its professionalism.

An alternate association, the American Society of Plastic and Reconstructive Surgeons, was formed in 1931 after Jacques W. Maliniac (1889–1976) was rejected from joining the American Association of Oral and Plastic Surgeons. Membership in the AAOPS was dependent on having both a medical and a dental degree and limited its membership to 40. To be a member of the AAOPS required nominations from those within the group and, despite Maliniac's excellent reputation as a surgeon who had cared for the Balkan soldiers during World War I, he could not get accepted. In 1925, he went into private practice. In 1930, the commissioner of hospitals in New York City, Dr. William Greefe, funded the creation of a city-run clinic to assist people who had been severely disfigured. Maliniac assisted in the plans for this public service. The idea was to provide plastic surgery to people who had suffered at the hands of quacks, and patients who had consulted "beauty specialists" and received faulty treatment. Most of these people were from a lower-middle-class socioeconomic bracket and had neither the education to discriminate between an ethical physician and a charlatan nor the money to afford a legitimate doctor. Maliniac's group initially consisted of doctors from the northeast United States and grew to include the specialist

from the entire country. International membership included correspond-
ing members from London, France, Germany, Austria, and Italy. Maliniac was aware that it was important to acknowledge the psychiatric
component of any patient, before and after surgery. The original membership was composed of board-certified otolaryngologists, including
Gillies, and an ophthalmologist who had been excluded from the AAPS.

By this time, a number of other professional plastic surgery societies
had organized. During the 1950s and 1960s, Dean Lierle was the secretary
of the American Board of Otolaryngology. He required the students in his
residency program to take full facial plastic surgery training during their
tenure. Not everyone in otolaryngology endorsed the concept. Although
many practitioners had performed surgery to move ear tissues, excise met-
astatic tumors, repair congenital deformities, or perform other operations
that resulted in an improvement in appearance to their patients, they were
ambivalent regarding the value of cosmetic surgery for itself.

The American Association of Plastic Surgeons and the American Society
of Plastic and Reconstructive Surgeons produced a journal after World War II,
Plastic and Reconstructive Surgery. Then, in 1999, the association changed
its name again, this time to the American Society of Plastic Surgeons. When
the original journal *Plastic and Reconstructive Surgery* was published in
1946, its editorial policy was not to reject articles that focused exclusively on
cosmetic procedures. It is now the official journal of the American Society of
Plastic Surgeons, and its contents remain largely dedicated to repairs of defects caused by cancers, radiation, wounds, or congenital defects.

Similarly, the British Association of Plastic Surgeons was founded in 1946
with the purpose of relieving sickness and protecting and preserving public
health by the promotion and development of plastic surgery. The aim of the
association was to advance education in all aspects of plastic surgery. Their
journal name, originally the *British Journal of Plastic Surgery,* was changed
to the *Journal of Plastic, Reconstructive and Aesthetic Surgery* in 2006.

Currently, there are journals published by a variety of sources, some
peer reviewed, and others less academic. In prestigious professional journals, such as *Lancet* and the *New England Journal of Medicine*, there are
standards that authors must meet. Names in the masthead are usually well-
known, established individuals in the field. The "Aims and Scope" of each
journal outlines the types of articles that are appropriate. Many prosthesis
and drug companies produce publications that follow the format of journals with typefaces, columns, and sidebars, but they are really just advertisements for their products.

REFERENCE

Simons, Robert L. n.d. "About Us." http://www.abfprs.org/about/history.cfm.

SECTION II

CHAPTER 9

Introduction and Overview

The miraculous transformations that modern surgery allows are not without controversy. Plastic surgery's 20th-century major achievements and goals arose during wartime and the need to restore function to a soldier's limb, hand, or face. Morbidity varied inversely with mortality because fewer deaths meant more injuries and trauma to the living; so, although penicillin and sulfa could fight infection, the remaining danger was disfigurement, crippling, or amputation. When facial features were involved, the damage was horrendous: jaws were shattered, noses, ears, eyes, and mouths destroyed. Facial trauma was perhaps the worst because, in addition to interfering with essential physiology for survival such as eating, vision, hearing, and breathing, the psychological aspect of identity was severely compromised.

During World War I, facial prosthetic tin masks were fashioned by sculptors in Paris and London to hide disfigurement or substitute missing eyes, noses, ears, and jaws (Feo 2007, 17). This was not a new solution to a problem; interesting prosthetics had been used in non-wartime for hundreds of years prior, to hide facial tissue destruction caused by syphilis or other injuries. However, those masks were a ready-made solution for the massive numbers of individuals returned from the war because so many men suffered from head, neck, and facial injuries. Unfortunately, plastic surgery technology lagged behind weapon technology: more sophisticated weapons produced more challenging wounds. Paradoxically, the machinery of war that was so dreadful provided a positive side, an ever-growing laboratory for the emerging plastic surgeons. Huge tissue defects required repair and grafts. Not since the time of Tagliacozzi's repairs from vicious sword fights or adulterous husbands had there been such a demand for rhinoplasties.

THE HUMAN FACE HAS A SPECIAL SIGNIFICANCE

Both figuratively and literally, one does not want to lose face and, in addition to identity, the face has a social meaning. Since early beliefs about disease, disfigurement, or birthmarks were related to religion and God's punishment for sin; a mask that hid a problem communicated a negative message about that person (i.e., did something was wrong). And, in the absence of blatant proof of being in God's disfavor, even a face without blemish or injury had certain characteristics that signified class, status, morality, breeding, or criminality. The Italian scientist Caesar Lombroso developed a peculiar theory that criminals were more closely related to apes than were noncriminals, and one could predict criminal behavior from an apish appearance. A weak chin, a high forehead, a large nose, and a series of images with explanations demonstrated that physiognomy was associated with personality traits. Napoleon allegedly said that when he required a man for head work, he always took one with a big nose, because a long nose and a good head are inseparable (Holden 1950, 60). Since the time of Galen and his humoral scheme connecting personality traits (phlegmatic, sanguine, melancholic, and choleric) with particular body fluids (black bile, blood, mucus, and yellow bile), authors, such as the 19th-century embryologist C. R. Stockard, have hypothesized connections between the two. Pierre Abraham found a relationship between physiognomy and the way that movie directors typecast their actors and actresses; Claude Sigaud (1862–1921), a French physician, wrote about how physiology affected personality (Holden 1950, 61). The anthropologist, William H. Sheldon, published *Atlas of Men* (1954), a book with hundreds of photographs of men's bodies and a number scheme that classified their personality traits according to their body type: mesomorph, ectomorph, and endomorph. It is not surprising that body shape, size, and appearance are so important to individuals seeking plastic surgery, because these beliefs and values are part of our cultural heritage. Despite the unscientific nature of any of these "scientific studies," people still associate a "weak chin" with dishonesty, a "strong jaw" with hypermasculinity, or a "high forehead" with superior intelligence.

NORMALIZING SURGERY

Plastic surgery was meant to normalize, to restore to the previous well-being state of health that individuals enjoyed prior to wartime. However, other applications were soon realized in the civilian population. Children were able to benefit from the strides made by these early surgeons in areas such as plastic surgery to repair birth defects such as cleft palate and cleft lip, asymmetrical faces, ears that stuck out too far or scar revisions from severe burns. Then, with the advent of women's liberation and the sexual revolution, an entire industry developed and gained acceptance (i.e., plastic surgery for esthetic and cosmetic purposes). Instead of coming from a damaged or mutilated perspective, the patient now desired to look younger, more beautiful, thinner, or less ethnic. The growth of plastic surgery was a bit like the chicken and egg paradox: did patients create the need for new procedures or did the new procedures attract an ever-growing number of patients? Regardless of what came first, the boundary between necessary and elective surgery blurred as a culture that focused on appearance grew more dependent on the medical profession and technology to create perfect faces and bodies.

STANDARDS OF BEAUTY

At first, this medical industry was primarily marketed to the affluent and *nouveau riche*. However, just as the standard of beauty changed from the first wave of immigration until the present, values continued to influence ideals. The pug nose, once the stigma associated with a working-class, alcohol-indulging immigrant in the 1920s, changed into a desirable facial feature in the 1950s. Large breasts in the 1950s were no longer in vogue (or in *Vogue*) in the 1960s and 1970s, after a model named Twiggy came to represent the healthy, active, sexy young woman. Breast-reduction mammoplasty was performed on women whose pendulous breasts created painful shoulder and back problems, and on younger women who desired to model themselves after the new androgynous, slim, or boyish body. Women who had nursed their children long periods of time, lost weight, or simply aged, often had breasts that lost volume and sagged, referred to as "pancake breasts." Those women could undergo a new procedure using a spiral flap.

Since many plastic surgery procedures had been limited by materials and technology; the chemical industry was called on to develop safe materials that would not deform, decompose, or cause abscesses. These materials were just as essential to the new specialists as good training in surgical techniques. Much controversy ensued as a result of using these materials. Silicone injections were outright dangerous because the silicone migrated, leaving lumps and unsightly body contours. After implants were invented, some of these ruptured, while others formed fibrous adhesions that had to be broken up. The FDA (Federal Drug Administration), CDC (Center for Disease Control), and NAS (National Academy of Science) became involved in a more than 20-year ongoing public health issue.

Baby Boomers embraced running, working out, physical fitness, yoga, and dance as an expression of new social freedoms. With those activities, the body became the focus of social acceptability. Men and women were determined to improve on nature if nature failed to endow them with enough flesh in the right place. If a man couldn't build enough bulk in his calves with exercise, a gastrocnemius implant would suffice. If a woman didn't have enough cleavage, breast implants could solve that. Multiparous women demanded tummy tucks (abdominoplasties) to repair the stretched stomach muscles resulting from numerous pregnancies.

CAVEAT EMPTOR

As each new cosmetic or reconstructive procedure appeared, patients flocked to receive them with little fear or caution. Liposuction, Botox, facelifts, and cosmetic procedures were so much in demand that clinics opened solely to accommodate that demand. With ubiquitous locations came a multiplicity of issues. The psychiatric patient with a body dysmorphic disorder (BDD) found an ideal focus for his or her self-perception problem. BDD is "a distressing and impairing preoccupation with a nonexistent or sight defect in appearance" (Phillips et al. 2001, 504). If a woman couldn't find one physician who would perform a revision of a surgery or create abnormally large breasts, she could find another physician who would. The more severe the BDD, the less often surgery "fixed" the imagined problem. In fact, in one study, the majority of patients who received nonpsychiatric treatments (meaning plastic surgery to "fix" the psychiatric problem) were not benefited by them. Men were refused plastic surgery more often than were women. Perhaps if more women had been evaluated more stringently regarding their psychological status, there would have been fewer dissatisfied patients. Michael Jackson, the high profile singer/ entertainer, was not refused surgery and his destructive cycle of surgeries is discussed in the chapter on ethnicity.

NEEDS VERSUS WANTS

Research in embryology led to better understanding of cleft palate formation. New technologies in photography allowed for television transmission of surgical procedures and more physicians could benefit from distance learning. At the same time, the lack of new technologies presented challenges to military surgeons in Vietnam. Working in this Asian country with few resources and limited resources created an additional problem for the indigenous people, because the majority of American surgeons were surgical residents, dedicated but often inexperienced and without supervision. Operations were performed on military, civilian, and pediatric patients, many of whom were "the enemy" until they had been injured.

The human body itself is "plastic." From birth to death, cultural modifications change the individual's appearance to fit a particular normative consensus. However, the variability from country to country demonstrates that there is no cross-cultural real standard of how the human body should look. For example, Western cultures differ in appearance from African, Middle Eastern, or Asian cultures, although globalization has changed some of the former differences. Our genes combine and recombine to make us tall, short, robust, slender, pudgy, or wiry. In fact, that diversity and variability is what keeps any species from extinction. Every culture chooses how to modify the bodies of its people as a way to mark their membership. Tattoos, perforations, circumcisions, scarification, and piercing are a few of the ways that people inscribe themselves with the symbols of their culture. Paradoxically, the concepts of "race" and "gender" are just as variable. One assumes that these aspects of human difference are carved in stone and "givens." However, race and gender are cultural constructs, malleable and often self-assigned. Individuals can choose from an infinite repertoire of behaviors and procedures to conform to an individualistic personal ideal, a model, perhaps different than either parent. Plastic surgery is available to change or modify almost every body part.

ETHNICITY

Race, in most cases, is confused with ethnicity. There is only one race, the human race. However since people live in various geographic areas and tend to intermarry among their own (or used to), people from the same area share a similar appearance. At one time, biology books showed pictures of people from all over the world as distinct races. Toward the middle of the 20th century, the number of races dwindled until there were three: negroid, mongoloid, and caucasoid. The problem with the category of race was that it was used to associate mental, psychological, and moral traits with physical appearance. This characterization was known as racism and its most extreme expression was in Germany with the concept of a superior race. In 1994 *The Bell Curve,* a book written about racial differences in intelligence, created controversy because of the authors' premises. Often, the concept of race was used interchangeably with ethnicity. And since most people are used to using the word race to describe cultural differences, it took a critical reader to recognize the confusion between the two terms. The difference between race and ethnicity is that race is biological and ethnicity is cultural. The designation of race is arbitrary. One can learn that some people in India with very dark skins are designated as belonging to the Caucasian "race" and that at one time in the United States, anyone with one relative as far back as a great-grandparent who was "Negro" was considered "Negro." Native Americans have been allowed to choose for themselves how much they identify with a racial group. At one time, like the "Negro," "American Indians" were considered "Indian" if they had any relative at all who was not Caucasian. The significant knowledge for the field of plastic surgery is that the surgeon cannot assume that all patients share the ideal model. For one reason, ideal models change; for another, not every ethnicity desires to look like white Anglo-Saxon Americans.

The desire to conform, paired with the parental desire to have their children look as normal as possible, presents a dilemma for the child born with Down syndrome. Should the typical features be obliterated with painful, expensive, and time-consuming surgery? At one time, these surgeries were recommended to lessen the imagined or potential harm from stares that a child might endure.

All these issues regarding choice to "normalize or not" hinge on an historic change toward modernity, diversity, and acceptance of differences that were once disparaged. The originator of the name Down syndrome was a British physician who, because of the ethnocentric beliefs of his time, believed that the "mongoloid race" was inferior in intelligence to the white races and first referred to these mentally challenged children as having mongolism. As anthropology developed into a social science rather than a Victorian armchair philosophy, prejudices and ideal human types were shown to be mere projections of the scientists' own belief systems rather than factual. Modern research has shown that intelligence is equally distributed in all cultures and has nothing to do with skin color, nose size, jaw shape, or head shape. And to reiterate what has been stated in other chapters, ideals of beauty change. It is certainly difficult to make an informed decision regarding surgery in the face of television shows such as *Nip/Tuck*. The radical changes are there because the patients shown are extreme examples of before and after. Before choosing to have plastic surgery, one would be wise to investigate the history of fashions, fads, and ideals, exactly why one wants to change a feature, what will result in one's life as a consequence, and if one wants to conform to a fad or simply look better to oneself in the mirror.

It seems as if every day there is a new procedure or way for plastic surgeons to alter the human body. As of the writing of this book, the names rhinoplasty (nose job), liposuction, abdominoplasty (tummy tuck), breast augmentation (boob job), facelift, Botox, and liposuction are surgeries that virtually everyone has heard of. A less familiar surgery, repair of hypospadias (when the urethra does not extend to the tip of the penis), has a cosmetic component but is mainly performed to normalize a child's penis and create a normal urinary stream. Hypospadias occurs 3–5 times out of every 10,000 male births. Some plastic surgery is reparative, such as scar revision, cleft palate and cleft lip repair, and skin transplants. Those procedures restore important functions such as eating, drinking, or movement (in the case of burns that left extensive scars, impeding mobility). Other surgeries are cosmetic; they change the way a person looks. Most of those are age related, although others change body contours by adding artificial prostheses or by subtracting tissue. The third category of plastic surgery combines restorative and cosmetic. In the case of the morbidly obese individual who wants to lose weight and look thinner, where is the boundary between cosmetic and function? Who decides what is too fat or too thin? What is the ideal? We think we know, but different people have different models of perfection. In fact, some people are obsessed with perfection and seek to remove the slightest imperfection. Others accept the aging process or their bodies the way they are, holding other values as more important than appearance.

For the purposes of this book, it is useful to list and briefly describe those surgeries that plastic surgeons perform. The list is by no means exhaustive, and by the time this book is published, there will be new techniques or technologies developed. However, so that the potential patient can make

Table 9.1 Plastic Surgery Procedures

Face	Rhytidectomy	A variety of procedures such as an endoscopic forehead lift, eyelid lift, or neck lift
	Anesthesia	General or IV sedation, depending on extent of surgery
	Time	2-4 hours or more
	Risks	Bleeding, infection, nerve injury, scarring, poor healing, change in hairline contour
	Recovery	Back to full normal activities in 3 weeks
	Cost	$7,500–$20,000
Eyelid	Blepharoplasty	Excess skin and fatty tissue are removed in either or both upper and lower eyelids. Scalpel or laser is used.
	Anesthesia	Local anesthesia with IV sedation is most often used
	Time	1–2 hours
	Risks	Infection, temporary blurred vision, lid tightness
	Recovery	Approximately 1 week
	Cost	$2,700–$5,200

(*Continued*)

Table 9.1 Plastic Surgery Procedures (*Continued*)

Forehead	Forehead/brow lift	Muscles and skin are tightened to give the forehead a smooth appearance and raise the eyebrows. Collagen injections fill out defects and Botox might be used to keep eyebrow muscles from contracting.
	Anesthesia	General and or local
	Time	1–2 hours
	Risks	Infection, nerve damage, bleeding
	Recovery	Minimal, same day
	Cost	$2,150–$4,300
Neck lift		Remove jowls, tighten loose muscles, remove fat. Redrape skin, improve jawline and correct double chin. An incision is made beneath the chin to allow for liposuction, liposculpture, and skin trimming. Submental lipectomy is performed so no scar will be obvious. Sometimes the incision is made behind the ear.
	Anesthesia	General and/or local with IV sedation
	Time	2–3 hours
	Risk	Infection, loss of sensation, scarring
	Recovery	1 week
	Cost	$4,000–$5,500
Chin, jaw and cheek implants		Incisions are made in natural crease lines externally or inside the mouth. Implants are placed inside the incisions and closedwith sutures. Sometimes, liposculpture or fat injections from patient's body are used.
	Anesthesia	General or local anesthesia with IV sedation
	Time	30 minutes to 2 hours
	Risk	Infection, hardening of scar tissue around the implant, shifting of the implant. Numbness and/or aching for a few days to 2 weeks. Chewing might be uncomfortable; mouth may feel stiff; swelling may last for 1–2 weeks; jaw implants may cause bruising.
	Cost	$2,000–$8,000

Table 9.1 Plastic Surgery Procedures (*Continued*)

Ear	Otoplasty	Large protruding ears, often on young children
	Anesthesia	General or local with IV sedation
	Time	2–3 hours
	Risk	Bleeding, infection, scarring, and uneven or mismatched ears
	Recovery	5–10 days for back to school or work; 1–2 months for full activities
	Cost	$3,000–$4,500
Lip	Plumping, lip lift	Collagen injections, Alloderm graft for plumping; for lip lift, skin is removed from the area between the upper lip and the nose. The incision is made at the base of the nose.
	Anesthesia	Local or IV sedation
	Risk	Swelling, bruising, allergic reaction, infection
	Recovery	Several days
	Cost	$2,000–$4,500
Mouth	Cleft lip/Cleft palate	"Cheiloplasty" refers to the repair of a cleft lip. A rotation advancement flap or a triangular flap method is used to correct a unilateral (one-sided) cleft lip. A palatoplasty closes the soft palate (roof of the mouth). This should be done before the child learns to speak. Then, when the child is between 1 year and 18 months of age, the hard palate is closed. The double-opposed Z-plasty technique normalizes the speech apparatus and does not effect jawbone growth. Sometimes a pharyngoplasty is performed to close the pharynx and nasopharynx, if speech is too nasal. This is done when either when the hard palate is repaired or when the child is in the early teens.
	Anesthesia	General, with local epinephrine to control bleeding
	Risk	As with any surgery, bleeding, postoperative infection, poor healing, irregular healing, problems with anesthesia, damage to deeper tissues

an informed choice before undergoing any procedure, the generalities are listed in Table 9.1.

REFERENCES

Feo, Katherine. 2007. "Invisibility: Memory, Masks and Masculinities in the Great War." *Journal of Design History* 20 (1): 17–27.

Holden, Harold M. 1950. *Noses.* Cleveland: The World Publishing Company.

Phillips, Katharine A., Jon Grant, Jason Siniscalchi, and Ralph Albertini. 2001. "Surgical and Nonpsychiatric Medical Treatment of Patients with Body Dysmorphic Disorder." *Psychosomatics* 42 (6): 504–10.

Sheldon, William. 1954. *Atlas of Men: A Guide for Somatotyping the Adult Male at All Ages.* New York: Gramercy Publishing Company.

CHAPTER 10

Informed Consent: Doctors and Patients at Risk

Making a decision to have any kind of a medical procedure is serious one and should take time. A person must research both the surgeon and the procedure. One of the most important considerations is the requirement that the physician be board certified. This means that he or she has performed a certain number of procedures that satisfied the credentialing requirements of the governing board. The doctor's assessment of the patient is equally important. The plastic surgeon must evaluate the emotional, psychological, physical, and health status of the potential patient before doing any procedure. From this extensive examination, a set of criteria are created to inform the patient about his or her risks or benefits should he or she decide to have the procedure. This information is referred to as "informed consent" and is written in a form that the patient will read and sign to indicate that he or she has understood the information.

RATIONALES FOR PLASTIC SURGERY

Patients go to plastic surgeons for a variety of reasons. Often they have been contemplating a cosmetic or esthetic procedure for a long time, and have finally decided to obtain a consultation. Others might have a congenital anomaly, been involved in an automobile accident, or been severely burned. A third group should not have plastic surgery: they are people who think that if only they had a smaller nose, or larger hips, or some other bodily alteration their life would change. Those people would be wise to get psychological counseling before undergoing surgery.

The number of cosmetic or esthetic procedures available increases each year and expands the possibilities for an individual to look younger or more beautiful. In 2010, the top four cosmetic surgical procedures were augmentation mammoplasty (breast augmentation), blepharoplasty (eyelid surgery), liposuction, and rhinoplasty (nose reshaping). There are television programs that glamorize plastic surgery so much that the specialty is trivialized to the point of appearing as mundane as a trip to the beauty parlor. The ease and simplicity of the production would lead one to believe that these surgeries are painless and without risk. However, any surgery has its caveats, particularly cosmetic or esthetic plastic surgery. When reconstructive or reparative surgery is performed on a traumatized, sick, or injured patient, that patient will improve or get well as a result of the operation. By contrast, esthetic plastic surgery is performed on normal or otherwise attractive individuals who are already healthy—in fact, must be in excellent health—and wish to go beyond normal or natural. Some patients state they want to try to improve on nature. Other reasons for wanting surgery will be discussed in Chapter 20, "Why Would Anyone Want to Do That?"

Physicians might show before-after pictures of similar cases or films of actual surgery. But no matter how many pictures are available, the patient should ask the doctor a number of questions. First and most important is if the surgeon is board certified. A board certification means that a doctor went beyond medical school and received specialty training. As part of that training the physician was required to perform a certain number of procedures either as an assistant or the primary operator. There are many kinds of board certifications and a board certified doctor in surgery is not the same as a board certified doctor in plastic surgery. If one is considering plastic surgery, one should not only look at the diplomas on the wall, but also carefully read them. A potential patient should take the time to look up any words that are unclear or not familiar. A person contemplating using a particular surgeon should ask the physician how many procedures he or she has performed on similar cases and how recently.

Body Dysmorphic Disorder

Likewise, a physician should question the patient regarding the requested alteration to make certain that the patient is choosing the right medical specialty for the defined problem. There is a psychiatric condition known as body dysmorphic disorder (BDD) that cripples a person's ability to realistically see one's image in a mirror. Patients seeking plastic surgery often have underlying psychological problems related to BDD or low self-esteem that could interfere with an acceptable result. In fact, those patients often continue to seek surgery after the initial procedure has been completed because they find another "defect" to correct. A patient with BDD might go from physician to physician until finding one who will agree to do the surgery. Unfortunately, a patient shopping for plastic surgeons who does not find an ethical doctor to perform the desired procedure often ends up at a plastic surgery clinic-type facility where standards are not as high as in a private-practice office. If that patient who has been refused surgery at one facility because of his or her psychological status is operated on at another, he or she is likely to be dissatisfied with the result. Since the problem is not physical but, rather, emotional or mental, plastic surgery will never help his or her image. And even though the low-cost clinics are in themselves risky for real reasons, the patient's complaints, regardless of their validity, will damage further the clinic's reputation. The plastic surgeon who can recognize a patient with BDD will at least save himself or herself aggravation and possibly an unjustified lawsuit. For that reason, not only do patients choose their doctors but doctors choose their patients. As a result of the surgery the patient should not expect radical life changes such as a new romantic partner or a drastic change in social status. To aspire to have such dramatic life improvements as a result of potential plastic surgery is unrealistic and usually such patients are not satisfied with their surgery, which they blame for other issues.

Other than those patients with BDD who seek plastic surgery as the key to happiness, a new love or a life-changing experience are patients who want a sex change or plastic surgery to make them look like a celebrity or, in the case of Michael Jackson, who ended up looking like a mutilated individual (Dull and West 1991, 58). Michael Jackson, the black icon of music and dance who died in 2009, underwent so many surgeries that he appeared to be a strange hybrid, with neither male nor female, African American or Caucasoid facial features. The psychiatrist Karl Menninger wrote about polysurgery and polysurgery addiction in the 1930s to describe a patient who continues to undergo surgery for such reasons as "secondary satisfactions of exhibitionism, passive submission to the surgeon, love and attention from the father" (Menninger 1934, 174). Although one cannot analyze the reasons for Michael Jackson's multiple surgeries, it is obvious that the series of operations and revisions left him deformed enough to require tissue from his ear to construct a new nose.

It is useful to ask the patient to articulate specifically what he or she would like to have done and why. Another question a physician should ask the patient is why she has chosen this particular time to have the procedure. By asking open-ended questions, the physician opens a dialog to help the patient explain to the physician the reasons behind seeking a consultation. Has the patient wanted to have this procedure only recently or has it been something that the patient has considered for a while? If the decision is only recent, it would be useful to find out if there was any event that escalated the need to have the surgery.

The physician should ask the patient why he or she has chosen a particular surgeon. Was there a particularly attractive ad? Or was the patient referred by a friend? Is this a second opinion? Often, a satisfied patient will recommend a particular plastic surgeon to a friend. This is good, because it demonstrates satisfaction, trust, and a positive attitude toward the doctor. In contrast to a healthy reason for wanting surgery, an unhappy or needy person might want plastic surgery as a way to gain attention from the physician or from others after the surgery is completed. Through these questions and the responses, the physician can evaluate whether the patient has realistic needs and expectations. Cosmetic or aesthetic plastic surgery differs from other types of surgery because the patient, rather than the physician, initiates the process.

THE INFORMED CONSENT FORM

In order to make certain that the patient understands the benefits and potential risks of the procedure, a form known as "Informed Consent" will be given to the patient to read and sign. According to the American Medical Association, the form must contain:

1. The patient's diagnosis;
2. The nature and purpose of the proposed treatment or procedure;
3. The risks and benefits of the proposed treatment or procedure;
4. Alternatives (regardless of their cost or the extent to which the treatment options are covered by health insurance);
5. The risks and benefits of the alternative treatment or procedure; and
6. The risks and benefits of not receiving or undergoing a treatment or procedure.

The patient should be given enough time to read and comprehend the information prior to signing it. The physician can offer assistance or ask whether the patient has any questions. If the patient does have questions, the physician should answer them, and continue to evaluate whether the patient understands everything in the disclaimer before moving on to the next step in the process. The Informed Consent form constitutes both an ethical obligation and a legal requirement. In addition to the signed informed consent form, many plastic surgeons require a pre-qualification psychological or psychiatric evaluation. The reason for this is to identify how much fantasy the potential patient is investing in the potential surgery. In 1988, more than 500,000 people had cosmetic surgery and that number only reflected procedures performed in hospitals. At that time, the American Society of Plastic and Reconstructive Surgeons (ASP&RS) estimated that 95 percent of the procedures were performed in the doctors' offices or in outpatient clinics, but it is difficult to accurately count the total number because of the growth of free-standing plastic surgery clinics. At that time, there were 2,660 active physician members of the American Society of Plastic and Reconstructive Surgeons.

If the patient is a consenting adult, where should the surgeon draw the line and not perform a particular procedure? Each physician can determine the limitations of his or her particular practice and inform the patient at that time. With the ubiquitous nature of the Internet, a person can find a plastic surgeon to do any procedure but that does not mean that the conditions will be ideal. In addition to finding the right physician, the patient must determine how much aftercare will be required and if the facility is certified by the proper medical overseers.

When a patient is younger than the age of consent, how does a doctor determine the validity of a parent's choice for a child? There is no doubt that a baby with cleft palate, harelip, or other facial defect that interferes with function requires a repair. Certainly ears that do not lie flat against the face might eventually cause a child to shy away from social contact because of ridicule. But a teenager's "hook" nose or large breasts could be more problematic to the parent than to the child, or vice versa. One must be aware of cultural dimensions of beauty and acceptability in a world of diverse social groups and standards.

Ambiguous Genitalia

Issues that have remained hidden from intensive public scrutiny are cases of children who are born with ambiguous genitalia whose parents made a decision to raise them as the opposite gender than their biological complement. Because the surgery altered their external genitalia so that it appeared "normal," and often deprived them of sexual pleasure, these children, now mature, are outraged that anyone had maimed them in such a way. They prefer that they had been left as they were born until they could make that decision for themselves. Other grown individuals feel that although they look like the sex of their genotype, they feel like a "woman in a man's body," or a "man in a woman's body." Those adults request sex-change surgery and will be required to undergo months of psychological counseling and evaluation prior to any operations. Although the first "sex change" operation was highly publicized when it was performed in Sweden in the 1950s, the techniques, materials, and technology are available in the United States where the transformation is no longer that unusual. The musician and co-developer of the Moog synthesizer, Walter Carlos, underwent a sex change in the 1970s to become Wendy Carlos. Her story and others are discussed in Chapter 19.

FINANCIAL CONSIDERATIONS

There are financial considerations, as well. A decision to undergo plastic surgical procedures is not so tidy, particularly when insurance companies and the IRS are ready to reject so many claims. Certain elective surgeries such as breast augmentation and facelifts, once tax deductible, were on a list of procedures that the 1990 Congress and Administration decided could not be used to help Americans improve their appearance. To add to the financial burden of the taxpayer, if the employer-sponsored health plan reimbursed the taxpayers for such a procedure, they would owe tax on the reimbursement received. At that time, a small liposuction procedure, which removed fat from the trunk and abdominal areas, cost $2,400 and the patient was able to receive a $792 tax credit. In order to qualify for any medical deduction, however, the total cost of medical expenses had to exceed 7.5 percent of the total income of the individual ("No New Tummies" 1990).

Informed consent involves multiple considerations on the part of the patient who seeks surgery and of the physician who consents to perform it. The following chapters discuss issues regarding the risks and benefits of plastic surgery.

REFERENCES

Dull, Diana, and Candace West. 1991. "Accounting for Cosmetic Surgery: The Accomplishment of Gender." *Social Problems* 38 (1): 54–70.

Menninger, K. A. 1934. "Polysurgery and Polysurgical Addiction." *Psychoanalyst Quarterly* 3: 173–99.

"No New Tummies: The Tax on Cosmetic Surgery." 1990. *New York Times,* November 17.

CHAPTER 11

Wartime Morality and Politics

In every war, morbidity and mortality vie for attention. Balanced against the cost of treatment, medical personnel must make decisions that appear to be no-win situations. As outlined in Section I, World War I gave birth to the plastic surgical techniques that came to be used during non-wartime for civilians. The types of injurious agents in the early 20th century, in addition to firearms, were various chemicals such as mustard gas, chlorine, phosgene, and vesicants, which produced burns and tissue destruction in those who did not die. Autografts and local flaps were performed on the war injured in World War I. During World War II, doctors and surgeons developed tube pedicles and forehead flaps. The technological advances in weaponry were significant during this time. Bombs, mines, and airborne and nuclear weapons were used and could kill larger numbers of people at one time. Unfortunately, this led to an increase in civilian and nonmilitary deaths and trauma. Each successive war led to a higher morbidity rate, because many of those who had survived did so because of life-saving advances in medicine, such as blood transfusions, antibiotics, and new medical technologies. Thus, an inverse ratio developed: the fewer the number of dead individuals, the greater would be the number of injured needing more immediate medical attention and follow-up care, physical therapy, and prosthetics.

GRAFTS

The first types of grafts, autografts, are transplants of skin from one part of the body to another. They proved to be superior to the original homografts that failed because they were transplanted from one individual to another. The reason for the graft failure was because the human immune system rejects materials that are foreign to it. In the case of an autograft, the tissue is from the person's own body. Many grafts were needed during wartime because of the extensive damage to the skin. In addition, ways to preserve tissue—so that if an individual had to be operated on in stages—some of that grafted skin could be preserved and prepared. The skin mesher, invented by Otto Lanz in 1908, was similar to a cheese slicer. It consisted of a board with a clamp and a knife attached to a bar, which could be moved to slice a very thin layer of skin. Skin could be cooled, freeze-dried, or preserved in saline solution for up to three weeks (Webster 1944). Homografts were performed on soldiers during World War II and the Korean War as temporary treatments until surgeons could obtain material from skin banks. But during wartime, freezing was not practical, so a new process similar to that used in food rations called freeze-drying was used and tissues could be stored for an indefinite length of time. Currently, scientists are working with regenerating and culturing new skin *in vitro*, meaning that the skin is taken from an individual and then prepared in a culture medium in a laboratory facility so that it will regenerate and produce a larger amount of tissue before it is grafted into the patient.

In order to avoid the urgency of wartime repairs in the face of inadequate training in plastic surgery, the Lackland Air Force Base in San Antonio, Texas, has started a unique program. The 59th Medical Wing provides all kinds of medical care to the men and women in the military, including reconstructive and cosmetic plastic surgery. The rationale behind the training is that most doctors in training do not see devastating war injuries unless they are involved in armed conflict. Therefore, by doing routine procedures on normal individuals, they get to reinforce the anatomical knowledge they learned in their first two years of medical school. Most physicians learn anatomy on cadavers, dead individuals who have been preserved in formalin. Their tissues are colorless and stiff, not pigmented like a living wounded individual would be. Most of the cadavers are people who died from natural causes, at an advanced age. Their bodies are not representative of the types of cases that these military surgeons will treat in the field. Training in anatomy in medical school is only for one year and future doctors work in teams. The advantage of being able to work with living, breathing people is that these surgeons learn the feel of normal warm tissue. Instead of preserved skin and muscle that is stiff and hard to cut, by operating on young, healthy individuals, surgeons can practice delicate techniques and do them routinely. Then, should an emergency occur, the surgeons will be more prepared for plastic procedures than without this training. These doctors perform reconstructive procedures and tummy tucks, between 60 and 80 each year, to keep current and knowledgeable in their technique ("Performing Cosmetic Plastic Surgery" 2011). During wartime, one of the most difficult issues for surgeons to face is that the majority of victims will be members of their peer group, younger people than those who were studied and practiced on when circumstances were normal. However, the peace-time experience they gain will help them enormously.

During the Vietnam War, high-velocity missiles produced gunshot wounds, fragment wounds, and "blast" wounds. More recently, our battles in Afghanistan and Iraqi led to similar wounds resulting from improvised explosive devices (IEDs). Those wounds destroy massive amounts of tissue and frequently get contaminated because of infused dirt and debris. During recent years, medical personnel have used triage and the staging of procedures. This process resulted in Two of three staged operations performed where the initial surgery took place in the field and later surgeries in medical facilities to repair, then reconstruct damaged tissues. The multitude of injuries provided a rich opportunity for new plastic surgeons to learn their skills under challenging conditions. However, some of the injuries were so horrendous that, in some cases, plastic surgery was not enough to create an acceptable result. Since the former protocol to use prosthetics in burn victims was gradually replaced by plastic surgery, those who were damaged too much to undergo surgery did not have as many options to obtain prosthetics.

PROSTHETICS

Older prostheses were heavy, awkward, and difficult to use. Fortunately, new reconstruction coordinated with prosthetics has none of the disadvantages of the 19th- and early 20th-century devices. The Maxillofacial Prosthetics Department at MacKown Dental Clinic builds prostheses for a variety of injured patients. Some are military personnel who were wounded in war; others are patients who have lost noses or ears because of cancer. Burn victims, amputees, and cancer patients are their three main demographics. A specialist known as an anaplastologist works with the patient to make a prosthesis that will be both functional and esthetically acceptable. Anaplastology is the "Art and science of restoring a malformed or absent part of the human body through artificial means" (Campbell 2010). The process involves stereolithography, a model made from 3-D epoxy and acrylic resin that creates a prototype based on the patient's own anatomy. From that model, the anaplastologist works to create whatever is needed to make that individual whole.

Sometimes, dental work and craniofacial implants are needed to restore a face. Prosthetics of old were artificial, heavy, and had to be attached to fake glasses to support them. The glasses had temples that hooked over the ears but when the person took the glasses off, the prosthesis came off with them. Modern prosthetics are made with silicone and resins that look and feel exactly like real tissue. They are attached by sophisticated means such as a titanium implant in bone that a magnet can attach to, or light weight strong adhesives that fasten the prosthesis directly to the head.

VOLUNTEERS AND NGOs

Despite the application of new techniques and the increased training for military surgeons, there remains a problem resulting from volunteer surgeons going overseas to third world or war-ravaged countries: the problem of charity plastic surgery. When clinics open in these pre-industrialized or poor countries, well-meaning residents and volunteers are often eager to travel to assist those in need. After the acute phase of the war is over, clinics expand their services to include congenital defects such as cleft palate. However, many of the surgical residents have no experience at all and are there to learn from the few board-qualified experienced physicians whom they accompany. Within a few weeks, the team leaves and the children are left to the indigenous physicians for aftercare and follow-up. If the local physicians have never cared for these kinds of surgical patients before, they may not have the necessary equipment for proper follow-up and care. In addition, certain countries suffer from gangs and guerilla warfare, groups of soldiers or other self-appointed military who terrorize their own people. They steal and appropriate food, antibiotics, and pain medicines for themselves. Thus, the children are left in situations where one must question: should developed countries help nations that have suffered from horrendous wars if the help cannot remain to provide aftercare? That is a problem only each volunteer medical and paramedical person must ask before going into a war torn country. One of the best resources to view is a film produced by Médecins Sans Frontiers (Doctors without Borders) called *Triage* (2008), where Dr. James Orbinski, the narrator, tells of his experiences in the 1990s in Somalia and Rwanda. This documentary follows Orbinski throughout the African countries where he tried to deliver health care to desperate people and discusses the problems related to politics interfering with humanitarian efforts.

REFERENCES

Campbell, Sue. 2010. "Air Force Dental Team Helps Patients 'Face' the World." *Air Force Print News Today.* www.af.mil/news/story.

"Performing Plastic Cosmetic Surgery Prepares Military Docs to Aid Wounded Soldiers." 2011. *The Plastic Surgery Channel.* www.theplasticsurgerychannel.com/breaking-news/performing—cosmetic.

Triage: Dr. James Orbinski's Humanitarian Dilemma. 2008. Sundance Films.

Webster, J. P. 1944. "Refrigerated Skin Grafts." *Annals of Surgery* 120: 421.

CHAPTER 12

Breast Reconstruction

Breast reconstruction is one of the most frequent procedures performed by board-certified plastic surgeons. The choice can be purely cosmetic or therapeutic, to restore the natural symmetry of a body that has been compromised by breast cancer. Until the invention of the silicone implant, the procedures used to augment or replace a breast were risky and, in some cases, resulted in more serious defects and scarring than prior to interventions. After a few years of routine restoration with silicone implants, a number of complaints started to trickle in to various government agencies. During the tumultuous years of the sexual revolution and women's liberation, women gained a voice and an audience as they forced dialog between consumer groups and the government. Women, previously silent and historically conditioned to believe the medical profession was beyond reproach, now demanded to know exactly what kinds of procedures were being performed and what materials were being implanted into their bodies. They insisted that they be informed about testing, safety, and longevity of any material, device, or substance that would be used to change their appearance. The government became involved and for the next 40 years, the controversies remained (and still remain) ongoing.

WHAT IS BREAST RECONSTRUCTION?

Breast reconstruction includes a variety of plastic surgery procedures that can be an option for women who have undergone mastectomy, or it can be an elective cosmetic surgical procedure for a healthy breast. Every woman who has experienced the physical and emotional trauma of breast cancer and the initial decisions regarding lumpectomy versus mastectomy, chemotherapy, radiation therapy, and adjuvant estrogen receptor medications faces additional challenges after the pathological tissue has been removed. Does she want to undergo breast reconstruction if it is possible?

If so, what type of implant or reconstruction is available? How close will the reconstructed breast match the intact breast? Will the intact breast be removed prophylactically and reconstructed so that both breasts will be identical? A recent trend over the past 20 years has been for the patient to be more involved in her choices of treatment, particularly since informed consent requires that the surgeon enumerate the alternatives, risks, benefits, or choice of no treatment and its risks and benefits. In 1990, there were 42,888 breast reconstructions performed by the members of the American Society of Plastic and Reconstructive Surgeons. This figure does not account for surgeries performed by nonmembers. The NIH estimated that 30 percent of women undergoing mastectomy will eventually have reconstruction surgery.

If the post-mastectomy patient decides to have reconstruction, there are a number of options available that allow more tissue conservation than previously possible. Armando Giuliano's article in the February 9, 2011, issue of the *Journal of the American Medical Association* reported that extensive surgery to remove all the lymph nodes that are involved with the cancer in a breast cancer patient is not necessary for all patients (Giuliano 2011). Previous surgery involved removal of the sentinel nodes in addition to axillary and any other local nodes. This required extensive tissue to be removed from under the arm, which caused two problems: swelling and edema of the arm because there was no longer drainage, and additional plastic surgery to correct the defect caused by the loss of the underlying tissue.

There are three basic types of reconstruction: implant, tissue flap (skin, fat, and muscle from the abdomen, back, or other areas of the body), or a combination of the two. The most common implant consists of an outer silicone shell filled with sterile saline (salt) solution. A silicone shell filled with silicone gel is another type of implant, but a series of complaints regarding leakage and potential health complications led to the development of the preferable saline-filled implant. There are alternative breast implants that are being used experimentally, but in order to obtain those, the patient must enroll in a clinical trial with a principle investigator. Often those studies are double-blinds, so that the patient does not know which kind of implant is being used.

If the patient opts for reconstruction, she must make an additional choice: immediate implant or reconstruction after initial healing has taken place. Immediate reconstruction is known as *one stage immediate breast reconstruction*. It is performed on the operating table by the plastic surgeon after the oncologic surgeon has completed the mastectomy. A *two-stage reconstruction* or *two-stage delayed reconstruction* is performed if the patient's skin and chest wall tissues are too tight and insufficient to accommodate an implant. When that occurs, a *tissue expander* (similar to a deflated balloon) is inserted under the skin and pectoral muscle. A tube that connects to a valve in the expander is used to inject saline and gradually inflate the implant at regular intervals until the breast implant is the size that the patient desires. After a period of four to six months, the skin will stretch enough to accommodate the "pumped up" implant. Depending on the elasticity of the skin, when it appears that enough tissue has been able to accommodate the expander, it can be removed and replaced with the permanent implant. Some surgeons prefer to leave the expander in place. When this done, the tubes are sealed and placed under the skin so that they do not show. Some expanders are left in place as the final implant. The advantage of this type of reconstruction is that the size can be made to exactly match the remaining intact breast. Another term for the *two-stage* reconstruction is sometimes called a *delayed-immediate reconstruction* because it allows choices. In certain cancers, the biopsy performed in the operating room is sent for a frozen section and stained so that the pathologist can look at it right away. If the surgeon determines that the patient should have radiation prior to reconstruction, than the incision is closed, the patient is scheduled for radiation, and the next stage is performed after the patient completes radiation therapy. If the slide is clear of cancer cells, then the surgeon can go ahead and perform whatever additional surgery is indicated. If a biopsy is performed in the operating room and it reveals that radiation is needed, the next steps may be delayed until after radiation therapy is complete. If radiation is not needed, the plastic surgeon can start right away with the tissue expander and the second surgery for reconstruction.

One deterrent to a decision regarding immediate reconstruction of a breast is that the prosthesis might prevent future detection of recurrent disease. Currently, the recurrence rate for breast cancer varies from 2 to 12 percent. Until the 1980s, the philosophy was to wait well after the mastectomy to reconstruct a breast. According to Langstein (2004, 672), "numerous reports have confirmed that breast reconstruction does not mask recurrence and that local relapses occur most commonly in the skin." Usually a patient who has undergone a mastectomy is followed very carefully in her postoperative time period. As in any surgery, there is initial recovery from anesthesia, stitch removal, wound care, and x-rays or MRIs to detect any changes other than normal healing. Since there is no breast tissue, a mammogram would not be necessary.

Another concern that pertains to waiting to reconstruct is that the postoperative complication rate could be higher. Some psychologists suggest that a patient might need to adjust to the idea that she has lost a significant body part that has a number of social and sexual connotations. The former idea that "mastectomy patients should 'live with the defect' for a period so that they would fully appreciate reconstructive efforts" (Langstein 2004,

672) seems cruel and unnecessary to the modern sensibility. However, a number of baby boomers have chosen to decline modification, because they feel it is unnatural. Others prefer to wait until they have had enough time to make a decision regarding reconstruction.

Reconstruction may not be as important to a slim, athletic, small-breasted woman whose profile will not change that much as a result of a mastectomy as it would be to a large-breasted woman who would look decidedly asymmetrical with only one breast. However, since reconstruction is an important decision, particularly if done immediately after the mastectomy, the patient and the doctor should discuss all the risks, benefits, and alternatives to reconstruction, regardless of breast size.

Since diagnostic and imaging techniques continue to be more accurate and sophisticated than previously, the detection of recurrent disease has not been impeded by immediate reconstruction of a breast. Certain studies have shown that the psychosocial benefit of immediate reconstruction reduces the emotional trauma of mastectomy. Postoperative complication rates have been proven to be 3–5 percent, approximately the same in either delayed or immediate reconstruction. In fact, there is less risk in undergoing the mastectomy and reconstruction during one surgical hospitalization than during two. The concomitant cost-savings would be from one rather than two admissions to the hospital; a shorter recuperative period; slighter anesthesia risk, because there would only be one surgical event; and fewer preoperative tests, x-rays, scans, and administrative paperwork. In 2008, the American Society of Plastic Surgeons (ASPS) created a registry for breast implants in collaboration with the FDA because of the occurrence of anaplastic large-cell lymphoma, a rare type of lymphoma developed by a few women who had received breast implants (Grady 2011). Although the lymphoma is not a type of breast cancer, and the incidence was 34 cases per 10 million since 1989, both agencies wanted to allay anxiety among potential patients. This type of lymphoma grows in the scar tissue that forms around the breast implant. To be on the side of caution, the FDA and the ASPS intend to establish and maintain an ongoing registry and collect data on breast implants to preclude the misinformation and false alarms that have been associated with breast implants (ASPS 2011).

Women who have not had breast cancer, but who have undergone extreme weight loss, breast-fed their children for long periods of time, or simply lost volume and skin elasticity in their breasts can sometimes have an alternative procedure to an implant called a spiral flap. Their breasts, described as "pancake," are reconstructed using fat and tissue from the abdomen or under the upper arm. The surgeon shapes it into a "breast mound and secures it with absorbable sutures into a tissue sheet that acts like a sling to hold the flap into position" (ASPS 2008). This technique is called liposculpture.

For a 20-year period beginning in 1984, silicon gel breast implants were banned by the FDA because a variety of autoimmune diseases were attributed to them. In November 2006, the FDA issued a news release regarding their approval for Allergan to market silicon gel-filled implants for women over the age of 22, and the ban was removed. That press release and an executive summary published by the National Academy of Science are excerpted in Section III, Primary Document 3. The authors of the executive report found five common complications associated with silicone gel implants: deflation, rupture, contracture (the formation of a fibrous tissue capsule around the implant), infection, hematoma, and pain. None of these complications were life threatening, although some required reoperation. The contracture problem was controlled by the creation of an implant shell with projections, known as texturing.

Breast reconstruction is such an important consideration in breast cancer patients that women should obtain as much information as possible. With regard to psychological satisfaction, one study that evaluated post-reconstruction surgery patients found that the women's attitudes were overwhelmingly positive (Rowland et al. 1993).

Any patient choosing to get breast reconstruction, immediate, delayed, or other (as in the case of sex-change operations) would be wise to consult with at least two physicians and research reputable sources of medical information such as the FDA, the National Cancer Institute (NCI), and the American Society of Plastic and Reconstructive Surgeons for brochures published especially for patients. Section III of this book contains primary documents with historic information about breast implants and safety.

REFERENCES AND FURTHER READING

ASPS. 2008. "Deflated 'Pancake Breasts' Restored after Pregnancy, Weight Loss, Aging." ASPS press release. www.plasticsurgery.org/Media/Press_Releases/ Deflated_Pancake_Breast.

ASPS. 2011. "ASPS Collaborates with FDA to Establish Breast Implant Registry." www.plasticsurgery.org/Media/Press_Releases/ASPS_Collaborates with FDA.

Bondurant, Stuart, Virginia Ernster, and Roger Herdman. n.d. *Silicone Breast Implants Committee on the Safety of Silicone Breast Implants Division of Health Promotion and Disease Prevention.* Washington, DC: Institute of Medicine, National Academy Press, National Academy of Sciences.

Cancer Statistics Review 1973–1989. 1992. NIH Publication #92–2789. Bethesda, MD: National Cancer Institute.

Corral, Claudio J., and Thomas A. Mustoe. 1996. "Controversy in Breast Reconstruction." *Surgical Clinics of North America* 76 (2): 309–26.

Grady, Denise. 2011. "Breast Implants Are Linked to Rare But Treatable Cancer, F.D.A. Finds." *New York Times,* January 26.

Giuliano, Armando E., Kelly K. Hunt, Karla V. Ballman, Peter D. Beitsch, Pat W. Whitworth, Peter W. Blumencranz, A. Marilyn Leitch, Sukamal Saha, Linda M. McCall, Monica Morrow. 2011. "Axillary Node Dissection vs. No Axillary Dissection in Women with Invasive Breast Cancer and Sentinel Node Metastasis: A Randomized Clinical Trial." *JAMA* 305 (6): 569–75.

Langstein, Howard N. 2004. Management of Recurrence in the Reconstructed Breast. In *Advanced Therapy of Breast Disease,* 2nd ed., ed. Gabriel N. Hortobagyi, S. Eva Singletary and Geoffrey L. Robb, 672–77. Hamilton, Ontario, Canada: B.C. Decker.

Rowland, J. H., J. C. Holland, T. Chaglassian, and D. Kinne. 1993. "Psychological Response to Breast Reconstruction: Expectations for and Impact on Postmastectomy Functioning." *Psychosomatics* 34: 241–50.

CHAPTER 13

Is Ethnicity Bad?

Ethnicity has often been conflated with "race" because both words imply that there is a group of people who share physical characteristics so distinctive that they should be regarded as different and deserving of an individual status, such as Italian, or German, or Indian. But wait, isn't Italian a nationality? Yes, Italian is a nationality, not a race, but what, then, is ethnicity? Ethnicity has to do with culture: food, clothing, habits, kinship rules, and language. Ethnicity also involves self-identification: a person of mixed ancestry can choose which culture or set of values to identify with. Not all people from a country look alike, especially in 2011. Immigration and emigration has lessened the rigid 19th-century categories and hierarchies that paired mental ability, personality, and atavism with a particular culture. This backward thinking held that every race or ethnic group had a physical characteristic which identified them as "the other." In America, as each wave of immigration changed the population demographic, upwardly mobile individuals chose to erase, blunt, or eradicate those features that made them distinct, in order to fit in. There was not too much that could be done about a change in skin color, but noses, lips, ears, and later cheeks, breasts, buttocks, and abdomens could be modified. In earlier chapters the Irish pug nose and the Jewish–Italian nose were discussed as the first examples that rhinoplasties were performed for esthetic and psychological reasons rather than out of functional necessity.

ETHNICITY AND CHOICE

Ethnicity is an interesting and confusing concept because peer or family pressure to remain in a group is often challenged by the desire to conform to the majority. However, during the radical years of social change in the 1960s and 1970s, "black is beautiful" gave rise to a new movement, one that valued and honored the African American cultural heritage.

The negroid features of kinky hair, plump lips, wide nasal breadth, and large buttocks were no longer perceived as negative. (The word *negroid* is an anthropological designation that refers to those facial physical features described previously.) During the 1960s, this community chose the term *black* to define themselves, but by the late 1980s, many black people chose to be referred to as African American. Sociocultural and some medical literature changed accordingly. Current medical literature uses African American instead of the terms "Negro," "colored," "negroid," or "black," which were formerly acceptable. Interestingly, the political organization NAACP (National Association for the Advancement of Colored People), never changed its acronym and states that it is an organization that supports the rights of ethnic minorities. For the purpose of these discussions, the terms African American and white will be used. Caucasian is not biologically or anthropologically correct because it refers to people from the Caucasus islands: the correct term would be "caucasoid." Physical anthropologists use the terms caucasoid, negroid, and mongoloid to describe certain skeletal features. But social scientists prefer Anglo or white instead of Caucasian, African American instead of negroid, and Asian instead of mongoloid or oriental. Those three terms were once considered races but there was so much physical variability within each group that the term "race" was meaningless. One only has to analyze Nazi Germany's criteria for race to recognize how truly dangerous using that term can be. They conflated hair color, eye color, skin color, nose shape, head measurements, and religion into one category that was actually political not biological. The entire categorization of peoples into races is confusing and most social scientists prefer to use the term *ethnicity*. Ethnicity is more than skin color, nose shape, lip thickness, or skull width. It is a more meaningful term because there is really only one race, the human race.

African American Populations

Until the late 1990s, cosmetic plastic surgery was viewed as unfavorable by African Americans, and was considered primarily a "white" choice. But this changed between 1997 and 2004 to reflect a 465 percent increase in the number of those who underwent procedures (Odunze et al. 2006, 1011). For those who did not want cosmetic plastic surgery, the primary reason was that a "change in their appearance would efface their ethnic identity" (Odunze et al. 2006, 1011). In addition, ethnicity was important in their choice of a plastic surgeon. Blepharoplasty (removal of bags under the eyes) is commonly performed on older patients, both black and white. One concern of African Americans was if they were going to have eyelid surgery, they wanted a surgeon who was of the same ethnicity and who understood their desire to retain their ethnicity, who would not make their eyes "too Caucasian." Unfortunately, at that time, there were not many African American plastic surgeons. Heeding these concerns, those Caucasian physicians studied the periorbital features that make the African American eye ethnically unique and learned from both morphological and measurable parameters that the African American eyelids shared certain characteristics with the Asian eyelid. When comparing youthful photographs of an individual with her current older appearance, that Asian similarity diminished with age. Once these African American women underwent blepharoplasty (eyelid surgery), some of that Asian eyelid feature was restored, which was acceptable. However, in contrast to what Caucasian patients desired, that is, "turning back the clock," African American women chose to have plastic surgery to accomplish a subtle change in looks and to feel better about themselves rather than look younger. Other African American women chose plastic surgery to "improve their social status as women who are racial minorities" (Kaw 1993, 78).

Younger African American patients have been able to undergo rhinoplasties, which have solved their potentially conflicting issues in a highly satisfactory manner, negotiating undesirable features while retaining ethnic identity and individuality. The esthetic ideal of these young people is totally different from that of Caucasians. Those aspects which they often want to change (in medical terms) in order to attain their ethnic ideal are: a wide depressed dorsum (highest part of the nose between the eyes), inadequate tip projection, poorly defined tip, excess alar flaring (width of the nostrils), diminished nasal length and height (short nose), an acute columellar-labial angle (area between upper lip and bottom of nose), and a low radix (upper part of the nose between the eyes). In other words, some of the distinctive African American features are self-perceived as merely exaggerated in those who seek to modify them.

No surgery is guaranteed to be free of complications, and both Caucasian and African American patients do experience them at the same rate, approximately 1 in every 20. However, distinctive complications experienced by African American patients are protracted edema, keloid formation (a type of raised scar), asymmetry at the alar base, nasal tip necrosis, and a problem described as "racial incongruity," a problem as a result of the surgery that results in a disproportion of facial features. The first two complications are related to skin and tissue. Most African Americans have thicker skin and when there are multiple incisions in the external skin, they require longer periods of healing. Keloid formation is typical of any scar formation, large or small, that African Americans experience. This factor should be taken into account by the patient before undergoing surgery and the patient should be made aware of all five potential problems in the informed consent consultation.

The other three problems are often summarized as caveats discussed in the medical literature for plastic surgeons. Nasal tip necrosis results from extensive alar base resections that continue to an area known as the alar groove; if the blood supply is cut off, then the tissue can no longer survive. Physicians are instructed to take extra care in preoperative planning and meticulous intraoperative hemostasis (bleeding). Postoperatively splinting the nose and using special tape prevents complications due to the prolonged healing time.

The high-profile case of Michael Jackson (1958–2009), the singer/performer, and his draconian demands to change his appearance illustrate two issues, physical and psychological. Jackson underwent his first plastic surgery procedure in 1979 when he was 21 and too many procedures to list after that, including a cartilage graft from his ear to his nose when one rhinoplasty revision became infected and destroyed so much tissue that he required an implant from another part of his body. His face changed so radically that it would be difficult for anyone who had formerly known him to recognize him. Not only did he change two typically African American features, such as the wide nasal bridge and epicanthic eye fold, but he had his facial skin bleached so that it would not be as dark as it had been. He seemed to be completely removing any suggestion that he was of caucasoid ancestry.

Asian American Populations

Eyelid surgery, known as oriental blepharoplasty, was performed as early as 1896 by Mikamo in Japan, and was popularized in the 1950s in Korea by Dr. David Ralph Millard. Millard was a commissioned Marine plastic surgeon who was chosen to remain behind after the end of the war to provide both medical relief and visible evidence of American good will in Asia. Millard had worked with Harold Delf Gillies during World War II, who had taught him reconstructive work for burns and pedicle flaps (Gillies and Millard 1957). However, Millard leaned toward perfecting aesthetic results beyond performing primary skin grafts, repair of cleft lip, and other wartime surgeries. One of his goals was to transform patients from "Oriental to Occidental," per their insistence. Millard felt that he was performing a humanitarian act by building a reputation for helping Asian people to become more acceptable to Americans. Because of the huge Anglo-American presence in Korea during the post-war period, and the fact that Millard had already built up a surgical community and trust in what he was doing, he was able facilitate this new aspiration. Millard's early work set the stage for what was became a Korean surgical community. In his 1955 article "Oriental Peregrinations" he writes of his translator who, in order to avoid being perceived as a "communist," opted to have eyelid surgery (Millard 1955). After World War II and Japan's involvement, followed by the Korean War, Asians were subject to distrust, which escalated to extreme suspicion and paranoia on the part of the American public regarding communism and Communist plots to take over the world. Therefore, in the perception of many Americans, "slant-eyed individuals" were associated with Communists (the "other") and with qualities that were associated with sneaky, untrustworthy, and unchristian. Millard later wrote how one identified patient, a young male translator who had worked in his clinic in Korea, no longer appeared "Oriental" and "after cartilage to nose and plastic to eyelids, the interpreter was mistaken for Mexican or Italian" (1955, 334). As an additional assurance that this surgery could remake an individual's acceptance in the anti-Communist world, he wrote that the translator became a Christian. These last two statements can only be appreciated if one understands the extreme fear and ethnocentrism of the 1950s.

Korea went on to become a hub of medical tourism, as did Korea, Japan, and Singapore. According to John DiMoia (2011), of the National University of Singapore, the ongoing dialog in Asia regarding double-eyelid surgery is not so much that patients want to become "Western" but more that they do not want to look "Asian." One of the choices of graduation presents now offered to teens in Korea is blepharoplasty. Plenty opt for this surgery instead of a new car.

As the Vietnam War came to a close, a new wave of Asian immigrants from Vietnam, Laos, and China arrived in the United States. By the 1980s, they had formed sizable Asian American populations. Many of these immigrants wished to change their faces and bodies to conform to what they felt were standard features of attractiveness: white America. Typical "caucasoid" characteristics were larger, rounder eyes, with more vertical height, modified by "double-eyelid surgery," large breasts, a heightened nasal bridge, and a modified nasal tip. In contrast to African American preferences, Asian Americans and Asians in Japan and other industrialized nations in Southeast Asia chose to modify their typical features and not preserve their ethnicity. The surgeries performed on Asian women (primarily) in addition to breast augmentation, rhinoplasty, and modification of the epicanthic eye fold are reduction malarplasty (an operation that makes cheekbones not so prominent) and mandibular reshaping (an operation that removes bone from the jaw to make it appear less "square").

LEG SURGERY

A concern of some overweight Asian women was the muscular definition in the calves of their legs. Total leg sculpture and liposuction, along with selective neurectomy, are procedures commonly performed in Taiwan (Tsai et al. 2009). A selective neurectomy involves destruction of the medial gastrocnemius muscle to minimize the calf size. Thus, although Asians and Asian Americans seek to Westernize their faces and upper bodies, they do not favor an athletic look to their legs. This Asian esthetic demonstrates a drastic cultural difference, because Americans often undergo plastic surgery and implants to the calf muscle to add bulk and definition to it. For those women who undergo selective medial neurectomy, the lateral muscle often hypertrophies (overgrows) to compensate for the loss of the medial muscle bundle, and the soleus can become damaged because of its proximity to the medial muscle bundle. This could cause a gait disturbance. Before and after photographs demonstrate that the patients are not able to rise up on the balls of their feet as high as prior to the surgery. As an interesting aside, manga comic books, graphic novels, and full-feature cartoons such as Miyazaki's *Spirited Away, Howl's Moving Castle, The Cat Returns,* and *My Neighbor Totoro,* while remaining consistent with Japanese culture, portray the humans with "round" eyes (Hirohi and Yoshimura 2010).

The attraction of plastic surgery to ethnically diverse individuals demonstrates that within any cultural group there will be individuals who seek to alter their appearance, either to make themselves look younger, "whiter," or more like others than like their own group. In addition, medical procedures, like high fashion and hairstyles, are fad-like and change every few decades. What was esthetically desirable at one point in history is no longer seen as attractive or beautiful in another, and what is the standard of beauty to one group is to be avoided by another. The difference between fashion and surgery is not as casual. Fashion and hairstyles are not permanent. They can be changed or reversed in moments or days. Plastic surgery is a medical procedure that requires invasive, intrusive, often destructive alterations in the human body that cannot be reversed. Surgery is painful and, therefore, requires anesthesia, which in itself is risky and has its own side effects. Shopping for a physician is quite different than making a decision about where to buy clothing, although some individuals might view it with the same attitude.

A study that analyzed the 40-year time span between 1966 and 2006 found the percentage of nonwhites in plastic surgery residents, fellows, and faculty in medical schools to be slightly more than 30 percent. In 2011, caucasoids still constitute 67 percent of all practitioners (Butler et al. 2009). Perhaps when this changes, minority patients will feel more comfortable in a health care environment that is more diverse. Knowing this, plastic surgeons can be sensitive to the preferences of these patients rather than to an assumed universal standard of beauty.

REFERENCES

Butler, Paris, Britt, L. D. and Michael T. Longaker. 2009. "Ethnic Diversity Remains Scarce in Academic Plastic and Reconstructive Surgery." *Plastic and Reconstructive Surgery* 123 (5): 1618–23.

DiMoia, John P. 2011. " 'Saving Faces' Eyelid Surgery and the South Korean Context, 1955–Present." Talk at the 2011 AAHM meeting, Philadelphia, Pennsylvania, April 28–May 1.

Gillies, Sir Harold, and David Ralph Millard. 1957. *The Principles and Art of Plastic Surgery: I.* Boston: Little Brown.

Hirohi, Toshitsugu, and Kotaro Yoshimura. 2010. "Vertical Enlargement of the Palpebral Aperture by Static Shortening of the Anterior and Posterior Lamellae of the Lower Eyelid: A Cosmetic Option for Asian Eyelids." *Surgical Clinics of North America* 76 (2): 309–26.

Kaw, Eugenia. 1993. "Medicalization of Racial Features: Asian American Women and Cosmetic Surgery." *Medical Anthropology Quarterly* 7 (1): 74–89.

Millard, David Ralph. 1955. "Oriental Peregrinations." *Plastic and Reconstructive Surgery* 16 (5): 319–36.

Odunze, Millicent, Reid, Russell, R., Yu, Maurice, and Julius W. Few 2006. "Periorbital Rejuvenation and the African American Patient: A Survey Approach." *Plastic and Reconstructive Surgery* 118 (4): 1011–18.

Tsai, Feng-Chou, Chien-Hao Chen, Chan-Yi Lin, and Li-Yung Ho. 2009. "Analysis of the Body Mass Index and Leg Profiles of Asian Women after Total Leg Sculpture." *Plastic and Reconstructive Surgery* 8: 643–50.

CHAPTER 14

Liposuction

Fat! A ubiquitous complaint. If only there were ways to eat all one wanted and not gain weight. That fantasy seemed to become a reality after surgeons such as Ivo Pitanguy in Brazil introduced the procedure of liposuction to the media (Huyssen 2003). This new technique replaced girdles, corsets, and stays; women threw away their baggy clothing and spread the news. Liposuction was promoted as a way to sculpt one's body and undo what years of bad nutrition had produced. Unfortunately, the instant success did not mean that people could continue their poor eating habits and it was certainly no substitute for prudent food intake or a diet to reach one's ideal body weight. Individuals prone to bodily dysmorphic syndrome identified every possible area for fat removal and still perseverated. Unscrupulous physicians, not board certified in plastic surgery, took short courses and opened up surgery centers, where they performed too many procedures with too few guidelines or restrictions on the candidate patients. Soon, patients were suing doctors due to unacceptable results. Others were dying from complications caused by combining multiple procedures—like tummy tucks combined with liposuction.

Whose fault were these errors: Unqualified doctors or unqualified patients?

REASONS FOR SURGICAL DISASTERS

Perhaps the answer lies in between. In clinics where the face-to-face interviews are conducted by paraprofessionals and not by the operating doctors, patients will undergo surgery without adequate screening. On the other hand, patients may so intensely desire surgery or liposuction that they lie about their medical history or drug use on the intake form. It is essential that a qualified physician conduct all plastic surgery procedures, from informed consent interview to postoperative care. This ensures that the patient has been evaluated for any possible complications from a pre-existing condition, such as emotional disabilities, diabetes, or gross obesity. Only then can one consent to the procedure.

WHAT IS LIPOSUCTION?

Liposuction is a procedure where subcutaneous fat is sucked out of a particular area of the body with a device similar to a small vacuum cleaner. A hand-held wand called a cannula, which is a little smaller in diameter than a pencil, is inserted into the "problem" area. It is attached to a tube that connects to a container that collects the removed fat. Areas of the body are marked with a pen to map out which areas will be removed. This is particularly important when performing liposuction on an extremely heavy individual, so that the result will be symmetrical. The cannula is placed in the deep underlying fat so that the surface or superficial fat remains to maintain a smooth appearance. Liposuction was started in France in the 1970s, using a large sharp cannula. The technique soon spread to the United States, and is now the most common esthetic plastic surgery procedure requested.

TUMESCENT LIPOSUCTION

In the 1980s, certain modifications were made to both the cannula and the technique to remove fat, so that it caused less trauma to the patient and greater ease of operation for the physician (Baj 1984). It is called *tumescent* or *wet tumescent* infusion. Saline solution with epinephrine, bicarbonate (and or triamolone, a steroid), and lidocaine are infiltrated into the area where fat is to be removed. The saline changes the tissue, making it easier to work with. When the skin over the fat appears very white, it demonstrates that the epinephrine has caused vasoconstriction. As a result of the infusion, the patient's fat becomes softer and easier for the suction machine to remove. The tools used are large spring-loaded syringes; a small, blunt-tipped cannula; roller pump machines; and hand-held syringes for small areas. When the cannula is introduced, it creates a tunnel, making suction easier and less traumatic. The epinephrine prevents bleeding and constricts the blood vessels. Previously, patients lost 20 milligrams of hemoglobin from bleeding during a liposuction procedure. When the tumescent technique was introduced, the average hemoglobin loss dropped to 9 milligrams per 100 grams of fat. Lidocaine diluted with bicarbonate provides the local anesthesia. Because the lidocaine is less concentrated, more can be used (Grazer and deJong 2000). According to Fortunato and McCullough (1998, 104), in a tumescent liposuction, 35–55 milligrams of this mixture per kilogram of body weight can be used without ill effect.

Triamolone is used to reduce inflammation. The physician uses less of his own muscle energy, as well.

One of the benefits of tumescent liposuction is that it can be used in conjunction with other procedures, such as facelifts (rhytidectomies). In neck liposuction, small incisions are made behind the ears and under the center of the chin. The surgeon pinches the skin to determine how much fat to remove and inserts the cannula under the skin, leaving 2 millimeters of subcutaneous tissue so that elasticity can be preserved. The prudent physician will remove a minimum of fat (about 50 ml) because in this area of the body, it is easier to come back later and remove more than it is to cause a large defect which will require a fat graft. The patient should remember that whenever fat is removed, if too much is removed, the remaining skin will not be youthful in appearance and may sag; therefore, after the liposuction, redundant skin will require additional surgery. Often skin in addition to fat will need to be removed.

Ultrasound-Assisted Liposuction (UAL)

Ultrasound-assisted liposuction (UAL) has been used in conjunction with tumescent liposuction for the past 10 years. The probes use sound waves to liquefy and break down fat before it is aspirated. Using ultrasound waves spares blood vessels, nerves, and lymphatics; it requires less pressure than traditional liposuction; therefore, bruising and bleeding are minimal. The surgeon can remove more fat with less trauma to surrounding tissue (Man and Faye 2002). When tumescent liposuction is used, IV sedation can be used instead of general anesthesia.

Other Considerations

When liposuction is used to contour the upper arm (suction brachioplasty), compression dressings must be applied immediately after the surgery. Such postoperative care should be considered prior to agreeing to such a procedure. So if a patient decides to have any kind of liposuction, they should ask about the type of aftercare required, the amount of pain to expect, and any potential complications that could occur.

As a minimum estimate, 293,000 lipoplasties were performed in 1996. It is the most common of all cosmetic plastic surgery procedures. The cost of a liposuction procedure, like any other, varies from geographic area to area and physician, part of the body and amount of fat removed. In 2002, one doctor charged from $2,700 to $6,000 or more, depending on the number of areas treated.

Fat is a necessary and important part of the human body and diet. It protects organs and gives shape and individuality to external appearances.

Without subcutaneous fat, humans would look very strange. Fats are necessary to store vitamins A, D, E, and K; they provide a concentrated source of energy to the body, and are necessary for the formation of essential natural steroids and hormones. Fats serve as insulation for the body from cold, preventing heat loss. However, a diet high in calories will produce more body fat than necessary, if the individual does not exercise or control intake. It is obvious when an individual is morbidly obese but what exactly is considered normal for humans? A generally accepted standard by the American Medical Association in the United States is that body fat should account for 20–27 percent of a woman's weight and 13–17 percent of a man's. Athletic individuals will have lower percentages and as one ages, the percentage increases. Overweight or obese individuals will have upward of 27 percent. Those individuals are not good candidates for liposuction, for a variety of reasons that will be discussed below.

Since percentage of body fat is not directly related to specific places on the body where fat accumulates, these foci are referred to as "problem areas." Fashion magazines and tabloids stress the negative aspects of fat by labeling areas such as "thunder thighs," "saddle bags," "love handles," "bat wings," "turkey wattle," "jowls," or "piano legs." In general, liposuction is most successfully accomplished when particular small areas are chosen for fat removal. Wise patients will not demand to have huge areas of fat removed, despite their dislike of their body. It is not uncommon for a patient to refused liposuction by an ethical physician, only to consult with a non–board-certified doctor, who will agree to perform the procedure. Unfortunately, since most of these doctors and facilities are not associated with a hospital—therefore not subject to peer review—the number of complications and fatalities goes unreported. Many fatalities occur during the one- or two-day postoperative period, often from residual hangover from anesthesia because the procedure was too lengthy.

Liposuction should not be used as a substitute for prudent dietary habits or to take the place of a weight loss program. The major risks such as scarring, bruising, bleeding, and burning are magnified in an overweight or obese patient, because there is so much tissue to remove. In addition, anyone undergoing surgery should obtain a physical examination by a general physician for clearance. Risk factors for any patient contemplating surgery are alcohol and tobacco or other substance dependencies; heart, blood vessel, or circulatory problems; and chronic emphysema or asthma, because they alter how the drugs used during surgery are metabolized. Serious complications and fatalities have been well documented in the medical literature when patients have not been completely honest and did not disclose information about their health or habits. A few of those complications are discussed here as a caveat to patients considering liposuction. The most common fatality documented during liposuction was pulmonary thromboembolism. This occurs when a blood clot impedes lung function and the patient dies.

Approximately 20 deaths per 100,000 (or 1 per 5,000 procedures) occur every year (Grazer and deJong 2000). Compared to the rate of motor vehicle fatalities at 16.4 per 100,000, the risk cannot be trivialized. In addition, this figure includes only board-certified physicians. One can only assume that a non–board-certified physician will have a higher ratio of complications and fatalities. Obviously, no matter how glossy the advertising, a patient shopping for a bargain will not benefit from choosing a physician who is not qualified to perform the surgery. There are a variety of weekend hands-on seminars for medical practitioners who are not plastic surgeons, through which they can earn a diploma stating that they have passed a course. This means that a nonphysician, such as a dentist, can obtain a certificate to hang on the wall, stating that he or she is qualified to perform whatever the seminar taught. An observant patient will examine all diplomas displayed on the wall and ask exactly what training it represents. Obviously, the weekend course does not substitute for the stringent training, requirements, rules, and regulations of the American Board of Plastic Surgeons.

CAVEAT EMPTOR

Unfortunately, liposuction clinics have become attractive commercial enterprises where naïve and uninformed patients take grave chances. At one Florida clinic that performs 29,000 plastic surgery procedures every year, there are 20 doctors who perform the surgery. That clinic was known to charge from one-third to one-half the fees that other less-advertised and better-supervised clinics charge. One of the physician's licenses had previously been suspended for three months and he was fined $10,000 because one of his patients almost died during liposuction (LaMendola 2011). That woman had to undergo two months of hospitalization for kidney and respiratory failure. She was a known diabetic whose condition put her at risk for any kind of surgery, and the plastic surgeon had failed to review her lab tests before operating on her. Because so many doctors work in commercial outpatient facilities, the physician who performed the surgery was not the same physician who conducted the intake interview. His reason for not knowing that she was diabetic is that he did not do the initial evaluation, and, thus, was unaware that the patient was diabetic. But, what possible excuse could he have for not reviewing her preoperative chart the day of surgery? That same physician had been sued six times for malpractice, lost his hospital privileges at a general hospital, and yet continued to perform surgeries at the outpatient center. The anesthesiologist who had assisted with another woman's surgery was working under probation with a suspended license because he had been involved with online prescriptions. At another low-cost clinic in south Florida that advertises on television, four patients in seven years died after undergoing surgery (Rab 2011).

WHEN FAT RETURNS

Until recently, no studies had been conducted on whether the fat removed by liposuction would return. It appeared that once a problem area had been liposuctioned, the fat would not return. However, a recent study on liposuction revealed that when liposuction removes fat from once place in the body, the body will regenerate fat in another part of the body (Kolata 2011). According to Teri L. Hernandez and Robert H. Eckel, two doctors at the University of Colorado, the human body will replace the fat it loses in another place a year after the liposuction (Hernandez et al. 2011). In other words, the body "defends" its fat. Genetically, everyone is endowed with a certain number of fat cells and when those are lost, the body replaces them. Despite this evidence, most patients who had elected to have fat removed from a particular place remained satisfied because the problem they consulted the plastic surgeon for had been solved.

REFERENCES

Baj, Pamela. 1984. "Lipo-Suction 'New Wave' Plastic Surgery." *American Journal of Nursing* (July): 892–93.

Fortunato, Nancymarie, and Susan M. McCullough. 1998. *Plastic and Reconstructive Surgery.* St. Louis: Mosby.

Grazer, Frederick M., and Rudolph H. de Jong. 2000. "Fatal Outcomes from Liposuction: Census Survey of Cosmetic Surgeons." *Plastic and Reconstructive Surgery* 105 (1): 436–46.

Hernandez, Teri L., John M. Kittelson, Christopher K. Law, Lawrence L. Ketch, Nicole R. Stob, Rachel C. Lindstrom, Ann Scherzinger, Elizabeth R. Stamm, and Robert H. Eckel. 2011. *Obesity. Fat Redistribution Following Suction Lipectomy: Defense of Body Fat and Patterns of Restoration* 19: 1388–95.

Huyssen, Antoine Hurtado, dir. 2003. *A Plastic Story.* New York: Icarus Films.

Kolata, Gina. 2011. "What Thighs Lose, Belly Finds." *New York Times,* May 1, WK5.

LaMendola, Bob. 2011. "Three Patients Died after Plastic Surgery Since '08." *Sun Sentinel* (Fort Lauderdale, FL), January 30, 1A.

Man, Daniel, and L. C. Faye. 2002. *The New Art of Man: Faces of Plastic Surgery.* Boca Raton, FL: BeautyArt Press.

Rab, Lisa. 2011. "Slice of Life." *New Times* (Broward-Palm Beach, FL), June 2–8, 9–15.

CHAPTER 15

Botox: A Good Use for a Bad Organism

Who would have thought that the most powerful exotoxin known, a neuro-toxin, produced by the bacterium *Clostridium botulinum*, could be modi-fied and controlled for use in esthetic surgery? The history of the disease, botulism, and its morbid symptoms of paralysis leading to fatal pulmonary arrest goes back to the 1870s, after contaminated sausage was ingested and caused food poisoning in humans. The illness was named botulism. In 1897 Emile Van Ermengen found that a bacterial toxin was related to botu-lism (Münchau and Bhatia 2000). Thus, for approximately 50 years, the germ was regarded as something to be avoided rather than cultivated. But from a medical standpoint, its evolution is interesting because, beginning in 1949, a form of botulinum started to be used for a number of strictly medical applications. Like many medical phenomena, creative applica-tions or innovations require a number of qualities in a researcher: experi-ence in a scientific field, awareness of other fields, and serendipity. In this case, the researcher(s) had to challenge a traditional paradigm and create a new application for a formerly uncontrollable substance.

ORIGINAL USES

In 1981, Alan Scott, an ophthalmologist, first used botulinum to correct *strabismus* (crossed eyes) and blepharospasm in humans after experiment-ing with other primates and mammals for a number of years. The treat-ment worked for only a few months and patients were required to return for more injections. However, the toxin that he was using had not been ap-proved by the FDA and he had to wait until Allergan manufactured a prod-uct that was in accordance with the FDA guidelines. In the early 1990s, other studies were done on the blocking effect of botulinum on another kind of spasm, one in the esophagus, part of the digestive apparatus.

BIOLOGY OF THE BUG

Clostridium botulinum consists of eight serotypes (subspecies), which produce seven toxins: A, B, C, D, E, F, and G (Jokli et al. 1992). The serotype commonly used by plastic surgeons is type A and is referred to as Botox, the brand name manufactured by the Allergan corporation. The toxin works by blocking the neurotransmitter, acetylcholine, a substance in the body that transmits nerve impulses to muscles. When the nerve is blocked, the muscle or muscles become paralyzed. The original uses were therapeutic in nature, to control pain, spasticity, tremor, eye problems, movement disorders, tics, multiple sclerosis, foot drop, and striated muscle pathology. Jost and Kohl (2001) listed 50 possible noncosmetic applications, including strabismus, cerebral palsy, cervical dystonia, blepharospasm, hemifacial spasm, spasmic torticollis, writer's cramp, tremors, tics, migraine headache, tension headache, achalasia, chronic anal fissure, hyperhidrosis, gustatory sweating, parkinsonism, myofascial pain, stroke, multiple sclerosis (MS) back pain, whiplash, and hypersalivation (Jost and Kohl 2001). All uses, medical and cosmetic, provided only temporary relief and required repeated application.

COSMETIC APPLICATIONS BEGIN

Botox was first used solely for cosmetic purposes by an ophthalmologist, Jean Carruthers, and her husband, a dermatologist, who had noted that when botulinum was used for blepharospasm, the frown lines between the eyes disappeared. They published their paper in the *Journal of Dermatological Surgery and Oncology* in 1992 (Carruthers and Carruthers 1992).

Cosmetic plastic surgeons found that by injecting small amounts of the toxin into facial areas where there is a tendency to form wrinkles, the skin smoothes out and the wrinkles disappear. The products marketed as Botox and Botox Cosmetic are manufactured by Allergan, the only company in the United States that is licensed by the FDA for cosmetic purposes. The forehead, areas around the eyes—referred to as "crows' feet"—and eyebrows are targeted as good areas for Botox. Although it is described as a safe procedure, like any foreign body, certain individuals could have allergic reactions or swelling. Botox Cosmetic recommends lower dosages than the Botox used for medical purposes but does not list some of the more serious side effects that are listed on the package for cosmetic use (FRAME). In the United Kingdom, Dysport is the brand name of type A toxin manufactured by Ipsen, Ltd. Elan Pharmaceuticals, Inc., manufactures a type B

Table 15.1 Preparations of Botulinum sold in the United States and Europe

Brand Name	Manufacturer	Generic Name	Serotype	Units per vial
Botox	Allergan	OnabotulinumtoxinA	A	100
MyBloc	Solstice Neuroscience	RimabotulinumtoxinB	B	75–125
NeuroBloc	Solstice Neuroscience	Rima	B	75–125
Dysport	Ipsen (France)	AbobotulinumtoxinA	A	40
Xeomin	Merz (Germany) Pharmaceuticals	IncobotulinumtoxinA	A	100

Note: One of the problems that face quality control in any clinic is that with the choices of toxin available, the operator must be extremely careful before using any produce because the dosages per cc differ between companies. If a clinic does not consistently order the same product because one company may be out of the product at the time, errors could result because each company markets a different number of units per vial.

toxin called MyoBloc that immediately produces a result but remains for a shorter amount of time and will need to be repeated (see Table 15.1).

CONSIDERATIONS

If a patient is taking antibiotics or any other medication, those drugs could either increase or reduce the potency of the injection. The effects of Botox used for cosmetic purposes, like Botox used for medical problems, are not permanent and within four to six months, the procedure must be repeated in order for the result to remain.

THE CRAZE

By 1998, the cosmetic application of the botulinum toxin for removal of facial lines had increased by 1,500 percent in the United States. Botox is the most popular noninvasive cosmetic procedure in the United States, estimated to have reached 3.8 million procedures in 2005. The procedure is so ubiquitous and accepted as routine that certain beauty salons have arranged with a plastic surgeon to sponsor a Botox party with champagne and hors d'oeuvres. They have a captive audience because those customers are already getting manicures, pedicures, or hairstyling. In one Boca Raton, Florida, salon, a sign-up sheet is prominently displayed at the cashier's desk, with a blurb about the plastic surgeon who will perform the procedures. In the back of the salon, near the changing room, is a huge glossy poster with photographs of elegant blond women sitting and smiling. The information for signing up is on that poster.

PROCEED WITH CAUTION

In the 20 years that Botox injections have been used, the most common side effects were temporary bruising, numbness at the injection site, nausea, headache, and flu-like symptoms (Miller 2011). However, when the botulinum toxin was used in nonplastic applications, severe side effects were documented which related to non-FDA approved uses and overdosing. After these adverse effects were noted, the FDA required the manufacturer to add a "black box" warning to its label (Mann 2009). This is the most stringent warning that any pharmaceutical can receive. Botox, when used according to the proper dosage, is safe for cosmetic surgery, provided the patient has no other health issues that could interfere.

In November 2004 in Fort Lauderdale, Florida, a chiropractor and his wife underwent what they believed were Botox injections from an acquaintance who operated a plastic surgery facility. Within 24 hours, they developed symptoms of weakness, dizziness, and double vision. Their symptoms escalated to total body paralysis and labored breathing. They were taken to a hospital and in the intensive care unit were put on ventilators so that they could breathe because their diaphragm muscles were paralyzed. The physician and his wife who supplied the substance were also taken ill and had to be hospitalized. Investigations by the CDC and Florida State health officials found the dosages to be excessive and from a batch of illegal nonapproved botulinum toxin. Two companies in Arizona, Powderz International and Toxin Research International, had supplied the clinic with unregulated toxins ("Doctor in Fake Botox Case" 2006).

CONTROVERSY RELATED TO ANIMAL TESTING

In addition to the issues of BDD patients seeking surgery to self-medicate emotional problems, and patients receiving the wrong serotype of *C. botulinum*, there is another issue raised by an organization whose goal is to protect animals from drastic medical experimentation. FRAME (an animal rights organization in the United Kingdom) has three concerns regarding the safety testing of *C. botulinum*. They feel that there has been no awareness of animal testing of Botox in the U.K. Traditionally, any drug is tested to provide information on an LD50 (lethal dose 50), meaning that if a particular substance is given to a group of animals, it will kill half (50%) of them. The LD50 for monkeys (species not stated) injected into a muscle is 40 units per kilogram of weight. Toxicity for humans is estimated to be similar. FRAME recommends that a more humane test be used, one that causes flaccid paralysis rather than death as its endpoint. They prefer that animals not be used at all, but that seems improbable, since the entire drug and pharmaceutical industry depends on the LD50 standard for determining toxicity in humans. In fact, the science of toxicology is based on the 16th-century physician Paracelsus, who stated: "The right dose differentiates a poison from a remedy."

Aging Is Inevitable

Although Botox can be dangerous to humans if used incorrectly, it has remained one of the most popular procedures performed by cosmetic plastic surgeons. The cost might be prohibitive to the average person, at approximately $140 per injection. However, to someone in the public eye whose facial appearance is extremely important, that cost would not be a concern. The real concern is the patient with BDD or who wants to deny the normal aging process, and cannot face that reality. If a Botox injection only lasts a few months and that patient is in her 30s when she gets her first injection, how long can she maintain a lifestyle that requires frequent injections (assuming that the physician allows such treatment to continue)? Such a patient probably has undergone a multiplicity of plastic surgeries and will continue to seek cosmetic fixes for psychological problems.

Any patient seeking frequent plastic surgery or Botox injections would be wise to reflect on his or her reasons for seeking repetitive procedures, particularly if the surgery did not solve the initial "problem."

References

Carruthers, Jean D., and Alastair Carruthers. 1992. "Treatment of Glabellar Frown Lines with *C. botulinum A* exotoxin." *Journal of Dermatological Surgery and Oncology* 18 (1): 17–21.

"Doctor in Fake Botox Case Sentenced to Three Years." 2006. *St. Petersburg Times,* January 26, 5B.

Jokli, Wolfgang K., Hilda P. Willett, D. Bernard Amos, and Catherine M. Wilfert. 1992. *Zinsser Microbiology,* 20th ed. Norwalk: Appleton and Lange.

Jost, Wolfgang H., and Andre Kohl. 2001. "Botulinum Toxin: Evidence-based Medicine Criteria in Rare Indications." *Journal of Neurology* 248: 39–44.

Mann, Denise. 2009. "Botox Gets Black Box Warning." http://www.yourplasticsurgeryguide.com/ injectables-and-fillers/botox-faq.htm.

Miller, Scott R. 2011. "Botox Injections—Benefits, Cost and Side Effects." http://www.yourplasticsurgeryguide.com/injectables-and-fillers/botox.htm.

Münchau, A., and K. P. Bhatia. 2000. "Uses of Botulinum Toxin Injection in Medicine Today." *British Medical Journal* 320: 161–65.

CHAPTER 16

Silicone and Other Implants

Silicon (Si) is a naturally occurring element that has been used for a multitude of applications. It is most commonly found as silicone dioxide (SiO_2). Long before computers and chips were fashioned from this substance, silicone was used to make ceramics, windows, drinking glasses, and, in certain medicines, dental abrasives and food powders. Later applications such as fiber optic cables and dental impression materials found silicone to be an excellent material. The baby boomer generation, with its "better things for better living through chemistry," embraced these advances in science, particularly medical science. Advances in plastic surgery, particularly cosmetic surgery, appealed to this generation more than ever. It is hard to imagine more uses for implants than there are at the present time; however, with improved microsurgical techniques, correction of joint defects and orthopaedic applications will likely be targeted for future silicone implants to correct the appearance of osteoarthritis deformities.

Although most people associate silicone implants with breast enhancement and facial plastic surgery, there are many other applications in medical science. Virtually every body part has been considered for potential repair, enlargement, or replacement with silicone. There are gels as well as solids used for implants. In the face and head, silicone implants have been used for brows, chins, cheeks, and ear cartilage replacement. In the musculoskeletal system, implants have been used for buttock and calf muscle enlargement. Bones and joints damaged by arthritis or other trauma have been modified with various types of silicone implants.

HISTORY

The history of breast replacement or enlargement begins in 1889 with Robert Gersuny, an Austrian plastic surgeon who experimented with paraffin injections. Although they caused tissue damage, disfigurement, infection, and sometimes death from fat embolism, paraffin continued to be used into the 1960s, often by unqualified practitioners. As a substitute, silicone, industrial silicone, developed during World War II became popular among Japanese prostitutes, who requested injections directly into the breast to attract the American soldiers who were stationed there. The custom spread to the United States, although the FDA never approved it. During the time period from the 1940s to the 1960s, nonindustrial silicone injections and polyvinyl sponges as implants were used for breast augmentation.

The 1960s was a time period of sexual liberation, but paradoxically, concurrent with the "I'm O.K., you're O.K." philosophy that deconstructed the ideal body, women started to reshape their bodies, most often getting breast augmentation. The notoriety of a San Francisco stripper, Carol Doda, and her huge breasts, enhanced by silicon injections, because so public a statement that such discussion and information was no longer private and secretive.

Then in 1962, Frank Gerow, a surgical resident in Houston, Texas, who routinely handled plastic IV bags and blood transfusion bags, came up with the idea that the problems caused by the sponges and other materials might be prevented if the breast implant could be contained in a bag similar to the IV saline bag. Together with his staff surgeon, Thomas Cronin and Dow Chemical (AKA Dow Corning), he developed the first fluid filled prosthesis in 1963. After experimenting with saline, they decided to use a more viscous material, silastic, a silicone gel compound. To preclude the possibility of migration, they used a piece of Dacron material as a patch that would attach the prosthesis to the chest wall. The prosthesis was successful in that it did not migrate but the Dacron patch caused an inflammatory reaction. As they modified the implant design, they were finally able to do away with patch. But there were problems with a hard fibrotic mass that developed around the prosthesis (encapsulation) much the same way an oyster forms a pearl from tissue irritation.

During the 1970s, a thinner bag was developed but this often ruptured or leaked. There was also some concern that the prosthesis prevented a radiologist's ability to detect changes in the breast. Since the implants were placed under the breast but over the chest wall muscle, plastic surgeons developed a new technique that made a pocket in the chest wall muscle which diminished the frequency of rupture, the encapsulation and the migration problems. Postoperative infections also decreased because there was no longer irritation to the ductal tissue.

Silicone implants are inert fist-sized bags that look like sandwich baggies filled with water. They are used to replace breast tissue that was removed because of cancer or to increase breast size in women who desire larger breasts. The issues and controversies regarding when or if to use them was discussed in Chapter 12, "Breast Reconstruction."

With the advent of plastics and the ability to create polymers in the mid-20th century, Ivalon (a polyethylene sac), Polystan (a relative of polyethelene strips wound into a ball), Etheron (a foam sponge related to polymethane), and Hydron (a substance related to methamethacrylate) were used at various times. with only temporary success because of problems with migration, irritation, and rejection.

Over the next 20 years, the number and types of silicone gel- and saline-filled implants became so popular that more than 1.9 million procedures had been performed. Since many prostheses were used to replace breasts that had been cancerous, often there was insufficient chest skin remaining to close over the additional material. Hilton Becker, a plastic surgeon in Boca Raton, Florida, developed a tissue expander to use in conjunction with the artificial breast. After the implant was placed, a tube was left in the body with a valve that could be accessed by the surgeon. As the patient's incision healed, the implant was gradually filled with liquid until the skin had an opportunity to adjust and stretch. When the breast was ideally filled, the tube and valve were removed, thus resulting in a safe and secure prosthesis.

In 1984, a series of complaints became public and the question of autoimmune disease with connective tissue disorders monopolized the arena of women's health issues. Since no definitive studies had been performed prior to the use of the implants, the manufacturers were criticized because no one had determined or questioned their safety or relationship to breast cancer, if any. On November 12, 1991, the General and Plastic Surgery Devices Panel (GPSDP) was assembled to meet in Gaithersburg, Maryland, to hear and review public testimony, and then make a recommendation to the FDA regarding silicone gel-filled implants. They heard complaints that varied from hair loss to fatigue. These were too nonspecific for the panel to reach a conclusion that connected silicone leakage into the body as the cause of systemic disease. However, in a later study, a silicone embolism was found to cause death when implants ruptured (Price, Schueler, and Perper 2006). Silicon injections, if composed of nonindustrial grades, could cause death as well when the material migrated. For a few years, breast implants using silicone gel were suspended. However, the GPSDP study concluded that although the implants served public interest in that they met a public health need (i.e., a woman's desire to replace cancerous breasts or to have a more idealized body), they should be considered experimental and no real danger was determined. But, "no real danger" did not mean that the implants were safe. It only meant that the agency could not find incontrovertible evidence that the implants caused disease, so, to be on the safe side, a de facto ban was announced and silicone implants were restricted for cosmetic purposes. Only women who had undergone mastectomies for cancer were allowed to receive them legally, which meant that if a patient insisted vociferously enough, she could obtain implants for cosmetic reasons. The report by the FDA regarding silicon breast implants is in Section III of this book.

In November 2006, newspapers published reports that the FDA's "ban" on implants had been lifted even though many women had gone against medical advice and were able to obtain them (Bridges n.d.). The FDA found that rupture was clearly documented in as high as 69 percent of the cases. It appears that although rupture was a predictable risk, systemic autoimmune disease could neither be proven as due to silicon implants or to other health factors that preexisted.

Since the entire history of silicone implants and breast augmentation with foreign materials has been plagued with failures and successes, a woman who decides to have silicone implants should follow good judgment in her choices (Stewart 1998). First, she should consult at least two board-certified plastic surgeons. If she has had one or two mastectomies, she has an additional concern, which would be a decision regarding immediate or future reconstruction. She should discuss the risks and benefits of the procedure and ask to see exactly what will be put in her body. There are a number of different techniques that secure implants to the body: some are under the chest muscle, others above it. She should ask herself how much her self-image is related to breast size and shape. American culture appears to be obsessed with breasts to an abnormal extent and that peculiarity needs to be examined (Gilman 1999; Latteier 1998). It is understandable that a cancer which requires removal of a body part that is part of one's gender identity, functional during childbearing years, and psychologically related to sexuality is a drastic incident. The diagnosis of cancer puts one in contact with one's mortality as well and decisions regarding that aspect of health care demands energy and other kinds of decision making.

Other than breast implants which most people associate with silicone, there is a variety of other uses for silicone compounds that plastic surgeons use. Silicons are used for joint replacements, implants to replace small bones in the hands and feet, silastic rods to act as tendon extensions to reconnect muscle to bone, and to fill other tissue defects. Unlike metal prostheses that fracture because of stress or have caused foreign body rejection, silicones have been relatively successful in restoration of function in body parts that are subjected to impact and pressure.

REFERENCES

Bridges, Andrew. n.d. "Silicone Breast Implant Ban Lifted after 14 Years." http://www.chron.com/disp/story.mpl/business/4343687.html.

Gilman, Sander. 1999. *Making the Body Beautiful: A Cultural History of Aesthetic Surgery.* Princeton, NJ: Princeton University Press.

Latteier, Carolyn. 1998. *Breasts: The Woman's Perspectiveon an American Obsession:* New York: Harrington Park Press.

Price, Eroston A., Harold Schueler, and Joshua A. Perper. 2006. "Massive Systemic Silicone Embolism: A Case Report and Review of Literature." *American Journal of Forensic Medicine and Pathology* 27 (2): 97–102.

Stewart, Mary. 1998. *Silicone Spills: Breast Implants on Trial.* Westport, CT: Praeger.

CHAPTER 17

Down Syndrome

Down syndrome (formerly referred to as Down's syndrome of mongolism trisomy 21) is a genetic defect where an individual has an additional 21st chromosome that results in mental retardation and a number of physical deformities ("Facts about Down Syndrome" n.d.). The appearance of a child with Down syndrome is remarkable for both physical and behavioral differences, varying from an individual with a severe inability to communicate to a high-functioning individual who responds appropriately to conversation and is only recognizable on close scrutiny of his or her physiognomy (epicanthic eyefold, thick neck). The life expectancy of a child born with Down's syndrome is approximately 55 years, less if the child has been institutionalized.

There are a number of plastic surgery reconstructions routinely performed on children with Down syndrome. These may include modifying the epicanthic eyefolds, performing a partial glossectomy to make the tongue smaller, inserting cheek implants, removing neck fat by liposuction, fixing the lower lip if it is turned down, and reducing the palpebral (eyelid) gap. The controversies involve whether or not it is ethical to "normalize" such a child if the procedures only result in appearance rather than an improvement in any functional aspect.

HISTORY

In the United States, approximately 1 out of every 1,000 child born will have Down syndrome. The incidence of Down syndrome increases with maternal age, as shown in Table 17.1.

The Down syndrome features are immediately apparent at birth. The facial profile will be flat, the eyes will have an upward slant, the neck will be short, and the ears may have a peculiar shape. Brushfield spots (white spots on the iris of the eye) are common and a single, deep transverse

Table 17.1 Incidence of Down Syndrome and Maternal Age

Mother's Age	Incidence of Down Syndrome
Under 30	< 1 in 1,000
30	1 in 900
35	1 in 400
36	1 in 300
37	1 in 230
38	1 in 180
39	1 in 135
40	1 in 105
42	1 in 60
44	1 in 35
46	1 in 20
48	1 in 16
49	1 in 12

crease (simian crease) on the palm of the hand is present. As the child grows, the skull will not develop normally, because the basilar suture (a place on the bottom on the skull where two bones fuse) fuses prematurely and the head shape is broader than it is long. The cheekbones are high, the eyes slanted, and there are prominent epicanthic eyefolds, so the individual's face appears Asian. There is hypoplasia (underdevelopment) of the nasal and facial bones and the eyes are wider apart than normal. There are extra skin folds in the neck. In some individuals, the ears are malformed. A Down syndrome child's lips might be thicker than usual or appear as if the lower lip is curled down, and the tongue is rough with fissures. The former pejorative appellation, "Mongoloid idiot" was coined because the person who first described the condition thought the children resembled people from Mongolia.

The syndrome was first medically described (and named after) John Langdon Down in 1866, but it was not until 1959 that the cause was discovered. In 1965, the World Health Organization dropped the term "mongolism" and adopted Down's syndrome as the appropriate nomenclature, nonetheless, some medical texts continue to use the older term. Later, the apostrophe and "s" were dropped in the United States but some literature in the United Kingdom uses Down's syndrome. Life expectancy varies depending on the type of care the individual receives, and in addition to being lower than 55 when institutionalized, is usually complicated by dementia similar to Alzheimer's during the fourth decade.

In 1998 a television program in the United Kingdom, *Changing Faces,* addressed the possibility that children with Down syndrome could benefit from plastic surgery that included bony reconstruction of the face. The claim of the proponents was that it would normalize the children and make them less subject to prejudice based on their appearance. In 2000, in the United States, one author published an article in the *Journal of Medical Ethics* and listed the procedures available to "normalize" the appearance of the face. That author felt that subjecting children with Down syndrome to major facial plastic surgery was mutilating and had no therapeutic benefit (Jones 2000). The British plastic surgeon R. R. Olbrisch (1982) believes that the facial appearance of a child presents a barrier between society and himself or herself, because the physical characteristics are tied to mental retardation and it is the intellectual deficiency that is the most disabling characteristic in Down syndrome. Therefore, he believes that if normalizing surgery is performed, it will minimize society's negative response to a child's appearance because the child will no longer have the physical appearance associated with a particular type of retarded person. Granted that in medicine most surgery is designed to cure a problem, improve function, or fix an abnormality, in the case of Down syndrome, nothing will be cured, and intellectual ability will not increase. However, if the surgery results in an easier life for the child and his parents by masking the child's disability, thus precluding negative glances or comments by strangers, then perhaps it is justified. Paradoxically, this could work against the child, because if he or she is perceived as "normal," then unusual behavior would not be tolerated or given latitude in view of the mental deficiency.

In certain studies, the parents of Down syndrome children have been pleased with the results of facial reconstruction (Olbrisch 1982). In another survey distributed to the parents of Down syndrome children, the parents were asked if they believed their child's appearance was perceived negatively by society and 72 percent of those surveyed indicated that it did not (Jones 2000). In a study with 50 adult patients who underwent a variety of procedures, such as partial glossectomy (reduction of the tongue), the authors found improved self-confidence in the majority of those patients because their speech had gotten better (Wexler et al. 1986). These studies are only three examples that demonstrate the complexity of the decision-making process that a child or patient with Down syndrome must address before undergoing facial reconstructive surgery. Certainly the medical benefits of any impairment dictate a therapeutic intervention. However, the National Down Syndrome Society does not recommend plastic surgery for cosmetic purposes. Their policy statement is included in the primary document section of this book.

REFERENCES

"Facts about Down Syndrome." n.d. NIH Eunice Kennedy Schriver National Institute of Child Health and Development. http://www.nichd.nih.gov/publica tions/ pubs/downsyndrome.cfm.

Jones, R. B. 2000. "Parental Consent to Cosmetic Facial Surgery in Down's Syndrome." *Journal of Medical Ethics* 26: 101–2.

Olbrisch, R. R. 1982. "Plastic Surgical Management of Children with Down Syndrome: Indications and Results." *British Journal of Plastic Surgery* 35: 195–200.

Wexler, Menachem-Ron, I. J. Peled, Y. Rand, Y. Mintzker, and R. Feuerstein.1986. "Rehabilitation of the Face in Patients with Down's Syndrome." *Journal of Plastic and Reconstructive Surgery* 77 (3): 383–93.

CHAPTER 18

Cleft Palate and Cleft Lip

HISTORY

A cleft palate (roof of the mouth) is a developmental defect that results in both functional and cosmetic defects. Often, a cleft palate is associated with a cleft lip, either on one side or both. During fetal development, the lip develops at approximately four to seven weeks and the cleft will form at that time. The opening extends into the nose and can be uni- or bilateral. In terms of frequency of birth defects in the United States, a study conducted by the CDC between 1999 and 2001 found that orofacial clefts are the most prevalent and that a cleft lip with or without a cleft palate is the fourth most common defect ("Improved National Prevalence Estimates" 2006). At that time, it was estimated that approximately 6,800 infants were affected every year, or 1 out of every 700 live births. Boys are affected twice as often as girls and the condition is more common in Asian children than in white and least common in blacks (Uhrich and Macklin 2001).

A cleft palate develops between the sixth to the ninth week of pregnancy. The cleft results from an incomplete closure of the palate. There are various degrees of severity, some that extend to the soft palate (in the back of the mouth) and others that are limited to the hard palate (front of the mouth). Since the palate protects the nose and airway from food and liquid, when a cleft palate is present, a child cannot drink or get adequate nutrition, because food and liquid go into nasal passages. Surgery to repair the cleft palate is usually performed in the first year of life. Repair to the cleft lip is done earlier, usually in the first few months of life; many surgeons will wait until the infant weighs 10 pounds and is 10 months old, so that certain facial muscles have had time to develop. However, the surgeries should be performed before the child begins to talk or tries to form meaningful words. Both conditions will require more surgeries later in life. Some of the additional surgeries could be placement of tubes

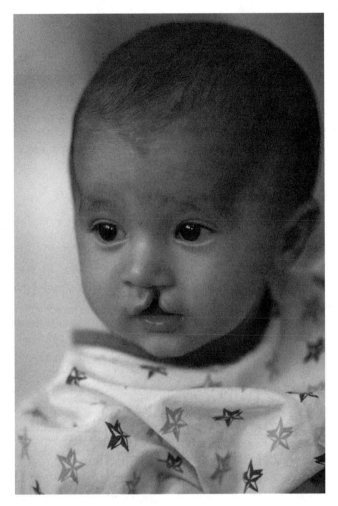

In this photo, taken September 22, 2009, Angel, 4 months old, waits for his cleft lip operation by the doctors of the Operation Smile team at the Institute for Reconstructive Plastic
Surgery in Guadalajara, Mexico. Operation Smile is a nonprofit medical service organization in which, since 1982, medical volunteers worldwide have treated more than 130,000
children born with cleft lips, cleft palates, and other facial deformities. (AP Photo/Carlos
Jasso)

to relieve fluid build-up in the Eustachian tubes, bone grafts to fill in the
alveolar ridge (gum line), secondary lip and nasal revisions, secondary
palate procedures and jaw surgery if the upper and lower jaws do not develop at the same rate. Since the teeth develop in the jaws and continue
to erupt throughout early childhood, a dentist and orthodontist probably
will be important adjuncts to the care of the child. Teeth are extremely
important to both appearance and nutritional function because they are

necessary for mastication and breaking food down into particles that are easily digestible.

Children who have already undergone surgeries and are aware that their appearance is different from their friends will benefit from as many "normalizing" procedures as possible. Many children go to a speech therapist because so much of word formation is compromised when the lips and mouth are modified. Since the nose is involved in certain cleft lip deformities, an ENT doctor might assist in any speech problems with a pronounced nasal quality. Since the children miss so much school during the important years of learning to read and write, they tend to be frequently diagnosed with learning disabilities. A learning disability is very different from a diagnosis of intellectual disability: there is no association of cleft lip, cleft palate, or both with intellectual disability.

The purpose of all these surgeries and therapies is to normalize the afflicted child as much as possible. There is no question that this type of plastic surgery is essential for both function and cosmetic purposes. That being said, an MSW social worker who was born with a cleft lip wrote an interesting narrative about her own experience (Aspinall 2006). Throughout her childhood, her grandmother often reassured her that her lip was "o.k." At the same time, the grandmother felt that she should console the child as if something was wrong with it, so the child received a mixed and confusing message. Aspinall (2006, 14) writes that she believes that appearance is "an issue for those of us who are anatomically different." However, she questions how and when a person's physical difference needs to be changed. She raises interesting questions regarding which differences are tolerated and why others are expected to change. If a physical difference is regarded as severe, she poses an interesting decision. She questions if it is really necessary to fix a physical difference instead of trying to designate a time to change it (i.e., *should* versus *when*). Additionally, she wonders if we should always try to make uncommon differences look more normal or even if an uncommon difference is a good thing.

Aspinall makes a point to differentiate the appearance of a person from the identity of a person. Fortunately for her, her education and professional training deconstructed the foundations of rejection, shame, and the psychological underpinnings of how society reacts to deformities, both to their own and to those of others. Her experience of living with the psychological pain of difference during childhood and her teen years by dealing with a variety of responses to her appearance (because she had scars) allowed her to understand her clients better than one who had not undergone those issues. When one of her three children was born with a unilateral cleft lip (she had a bilateral cleft lip), she was prepared as a parent and a social worker to deal with the anxiety of having a child undergo multiple surgeries and suffer painful recoveries. And although

she maintains her objectivity regarding the necessity of normalizing differences, she points out that "cleft surgery is not about preventing physical pain or a potential risk to life . . . it is primarily about protecting
your child (and yourself) from psychological pain" (Aspinall 2006, 24).
Aspinall did chose to have her youngest child undergo surgery for the
cleft lip, but when he was older (she didn't state how much older) he
expressed a desire to have the scar on his upper lip and his nostril fixed
so that it would be symmetric with the other. She involved him in the
consultation with the plastic surgeon and when he learned that some
cartilage from his ear would be used to fix his nostril, he chose not to
have the surgery because he did not want to experience any more pain.
Although Aspinall states that she believes that children should be involved in decisions that affect their health and well-being when they are
old enough to make an intelligent, informed decision, she does not say
how old that is nor does she say how old her son was when she involved
him in the decision. She does stress that it is important that parents do
not force their children into becoming something that they are not or do
not want to be.

Alternately, Kohn (2000) studied the patients and physicians in one
hospital in northern California, and found that the plastic surgery team
"emplotted" their communication to children. Their messages were that
the children were attractive and "worthy of attention and affection." They
wanted the children to know that the children's personhood was separate
from their facial anomaly: they may have had "imperfect" faces but they
were normal children (Kohn 2000).

At infancy there is very little controversy regarding the necessity to repair a cleft palate or cleft lip. Clearly, breathing, eating, and drinking are
compromised when a newborn has a defect that involves critical life processes. Since the repairs are not performed during only one operation, the
sequence of surgeries is a painful way to begin life. By the time a child
is 10, he or she may have undergone eight or nine procedures. The issues
involved address the question regarding informed consent on the part of
the child. How much of the decision should be the child's if additional surgeries are to be performed? On a global perspective, cleft palate remains a
problem for underdeveloped countries because of lack of caregiver training, hospital facilities, medicines, and technology. An issue regarding volunteer teams going to these countries focuses on how valuable foreign aid
is if sufficient postoperative care and support is not provided.

This is an issue regarding cleft palate repair that involves physician
training and third world or preindustrialized countries. Since cleft palate and lip are a worldwide occurrence, voluntary teams travel to remote
areas to perform plastic surgery. These are usually seasoned plastic surgeons and residents in training. In 2002, 20 individuals from the United

States went to a facility in Southeast Asia to operate on 98 children with cleft palates and cleft lips. They were allowed four of the five tables in that particular unnamed hospital for the plastic surgery, the fifth being for indigenous doctors to use in emergency situations. Although there were 20 surgeons, only 2 of them would have been qualified to perform the surgery in the United States because they were board certified. But, in a preindustrial or third-world country, residents were basically practicing on indigenous children. In one provincial Asian hospital, in 1999, two children died after a routine cleft palate repair because they were malnourished. In the United States, that death would have been considered malpractice because they would not have been prequalified or preapproved for surgery. Another problem is that visiting physicians do not stay long enough to take care of any complications that arose after surgery and follow up on the cases. When local surgeons perform the surgery, they are familiar with the patient: they know the family, the history, the interoperative procedures, and what kind of closure was chosen. But when surgeons from NGOs perform the surgery and leave, the local physicians are often at a loss to provide adequate aftercare if there are any complications, because they did not do or see the surgery and did not see what techniques, appliances, and implants of other devices may have been used. In one narrative, a team reportedly performed 135 operations in five days but then left. Although the initial results appear to be perfect, there are no figures for the complication rate. The surgeons who performed the surgery are now gone and, unless someone decides to do a statistical study on these 135 surgeries, there will be no follow-up information regarding complications or deaths. However, the local surgeons estimated that when amateur foreign plastic surgeons performed the cleft palate repairs, the complication rate was over 30 percent. That figure would be unacceptable in an American hospital. In one hospital when the local doctor volunteered to scrub in with the foreign visiting American surgeon, he was told that the surgeon preferred to work with his own nurse. This is a prime example of ethnocentrism and not what visiting foreigners should be communicating to people they allegedly intend to help.

Interestingly, one team working in Cambodia in 2002 estimated that the American cost for a cleft lip operation is $1,000 per child or $98,000 for the group of 98. By contrast, if a local doctor performs the surgery, the cost is $80. In Laos, in 2002, Handicap International sent a team who performed 95 operations in two weeks (Dupuis 2004). Obviously, the indigenous people could not have afforded those surgeries, either. The cost in U.S. dollars would have been $7,414 per procedure, but the surgery was free to the Laotians. Laotians accepted this generous offer by the foreign team to complete the surgeries because the cost would have been prohibitive for them otherwise, even at less than $100 per operation.

When expensive and complicated technology is donated to a community, it is important that the donor investigates if there is adequate infrastructure to support the equipment. For example, if a computer is provided, there must be sufficient bandwidth to make it functional; if an air conditioner is offered, there must be continuous electricity to keep it going. When drugs are donated, will they be used for the patients or will guerilla factions or other inappropriate individuals confiscate them for their own use? In countries where ongoing internecine conflicts cause upheavals, often equipment and pharmaceuticals are stolen before the patients ever get to benefit from them. It is important to evaluate the standards of living in a particular area to make certain that what is given to the people will be used by the people. The standards of living are so different in other countries that Americans are unable to predict, for example, that if they were to donate the most sophisticated piece of equipment, such as an air-conditioning unit, that the recipient might not have the fuel or power to operate it. The complications and issues regarding cleft palate operations performed by volunteer surgeons involve much more than the surgery itself and might not always be as altruistic as desired.

REFERENCES

Aspinall, Cassandra. 2006. "Do I Make You Uncomfortable? Reflections on Using Surgery to Reduce the Distress of Others." In *Surgically Shaping Children,* ed. Erik Parens, 13–28. Baltimore: Johns Hopkins University Press.

Dupuis, Christian. 2004. "Humanitarian Missions in the Third World: A Polite Dissent." *Plastic and Reconstructive Surgery* 113 (1): 433–35.

"Improved National Prevalence Estimates for 18 Selected Major Birth Defects— United States, 1999–2001." 2006. *Morbidity and Mortality Weekly Report* 54 (51/52): http://www.cdc.gov/mmwr/PDF/wk/mm5451.pdf.

Kohn, Abigail A. 2000. " 'Imperfect Angels': Narrative 'Emplotment' in the Medical Management of Children with Craniofacial Anomalies." *Medical Anthropology Quarterly* 14 (2): 202–23.

Uhrich, Kim S., and Amy L. Macklin. 2001. "Cleft Lip and Palate." *American Journal of Nursing* 101 (3): 24–29.

CHAPTER 19

Ambiguous Genitalia

Most people have been taught that male and female are two discrete sexes in humans and higher animals. Early in life, we were socialized to think in binary terms (either/or): boy or girl, man or woman, female or male. Then, in high school biology, we learned the word "reproduction," and the various ways other animals can reproduce. Not everyone needed two parents: a planarian cut in three could grow into two more planarians; a roundworm has both male and female sex organs. They can mate with any other worm and produce offspring. The word to describe their sexual anatomy was "hermaphroditic." Certain fish can change their sex to accommodate the necessary balance in the larger community if it lacked one or the other sex. Humans are allegedly either male or female, yet when there are exceptions, they are hidden and embarrassing exceptions. According to medical experts, until the late 20th century it was not possible for a "true" hermaphrodite to exist in the human species. Ambröise Paré, the famed surgeon who fashioned artificial hands for war veterans and who discovered the first logical treatment for burn victims, wrote a book showing all kinds of monsters, based on "supernatural occurrences," the result of "strange things." He described four types of hermaphrodites and "memorable stories of women who had degenerated into men." Although he postulated that the reasons for the anomalies were based on superstition, he was aware that such variations existed in the human species (Paré 1982).

HISTORY

There is pancultural evidence that individuals with abnormal genitalia existed at least since the 15th-century writings of Paré. In Colonial America, the 17th-century worldview regarded such births as proof that the mother held deformed or monstrous ideas. Religion played a prominent role in blaming the parent for any abnormalities in the newborn child.

It took more than 200 years before the sexual revolution of the 1960s made visible the possibility that human sexuality and its biological expression was variable and not clear-cut. Individuals were not identical in their orientation, just as they were not identical in the degree of femininity or masculinity they exhibited. Even skeletons show a gradation of types from male and female extremes at opposite ends of the pole, with a variety of intermediates.

The voices and dilemmas of certain in-between people entered the popular culture landscape with the publication of John Money's 1968 book *Sex Errors of the Body.* At that time, Money, a researcher from Johns Hopkins University, had been conducting studies and interviews with children and adults with various psychological conditions that involved sexual identity. Some of these individuals were male cross-dressers, content with their sex but having a desire to dress in women's clothing. Others were psychologically dissatisfied with their sex, expressing their discomfort as "a man in a woman's body" or "deep down inside, a woman in a man's body" (now referred to as transsexuals). Money adapted the term "gender" from linguistics to refer to the cultural constructs that shape an individual's psychosexual identity. Although the word had been used since 1825, it referred to inanimate objects. Money defined gender as a way that individuals conform to generally accepted roles within each culture that are clearly defined. For example, girls are "naturally" expected to be cooperative and obedient, like to play with dolls, like to read about romance, and have goals which focus on marriage and the family. Boys are expected to play with cars and trucks, be outgoing, daring, and court danger, and be interested in a profession or career.

The women's liberation movement of the 1960s attacked these stereotypes and tried to re-educate society by saying biology was not destiny and women, if not directed to play a female role in childhood, would not necessarily choose typically feminine activities. However, certain actions, behaviors, gestures, and paralanguage were clearly defined as either female or male. For example, a boy who walked and swung his hips was either exhibiting a parodic gait or referred to as "swishy." A girl who cut her hair very short and wore baggy clothing that camouflaged her breasts and small waist might be referred to as "butch." Those were choices that individuals could make without altering their bodies surgically. To summarize, gender was something that was fluid and cultural, taught and learned.

Sex versus Gender

Sex, on the other hand, is different from gender in that it is biological and given. A female has two X chromosomes, while a male has both an X and a Y chromosome. In the usual reproductive pattern, when a new individual is formed, it receives one gamete from each parent. If the male parent contributes the Y gamete, then the offspring will be male (XY); if the male parent contributes his X gamete, then the offspring will be female (XX). The dilemma that certain individuals face is that they were born with a genetic (genotypic) complement that does not outwardly match either the male or female phenotype. One definition of sex depends on four variables: chromosomal sex (female 46/XX or male 46/XY), Gonadal sex (the histological structure of the ovary or testis), external genitalia and body form, psychological sex. When all four criteria are present in the same individual, that individual is either male or female. If any of the four differ from the others, that individual is referred to as intersex. Approximately 1 in every 2,000 children is born with an intersex condition (Hillman 2008), an anomaly more common than cleft palate.

Intersex Individuals

Some, but not all, intersex individuals have associated medical conditions. The conditions that plastic surgeons usually treat are hypospadias, an opening under the penis for the urethra rather than at the tip; Androgen Insensitivity Syndrome (AIS); gonadal dysgenesis; and 5-alpha reductase deficiency. When the child has congenital adrenal hyperplasia (CAH), a female (XX) baby might appear to be male because she has an enlarged clitoris and fused labiae. Perhaps there are no external testicles, but internally the child has a uterus and ovaries. In a case such as this, the parents might consult a plastic surgeon to create a vagina. If the urethra is malpositioned, surgery will need to be performed to connect the urethra and perform a series of dilations until it is of normal diameter. Surgeries are done to reduce the size of the clitoris, although over the past 30 years, there has been a difference of opinion regarding this procedure. Unfortunately, these complex surgeries are so prohibitive in cost that parents who choose to have their children "normalized" usually go to a teaching hospital and spend long hours with physicians, therapists, and students.

Previous Decisions

Historically, if a baby was born with indeterminate genitalia, a team of specialists (e.g., urologist, plastic surgeon, endocrinologist, psychiatrist) was immediately consulted to talk to the parents in an effort to make a decision regarding sexual reassignment surgery. The assumption was that a child would not be able to deal with being different, but more importantly, the parents (and society) preferred to have a normal-looking child, even if sexual function would be compromised or impossible. Society, in general, has problems accepting any kind of diversity. This made logical sense when these surgeries first were performed. The 1960s research documented that a person's gender was socially constructed and if an individual were raised to be a girl, regardless of her biology, she would be a girl rather than what her biological makeup was. A qualification is that gender identity took place at a critical period in development, around the same time that language learning takes place, prior to 15 months of age. Unfortunately, the facts were not that simple.

The Turning Point

The case that attracted worldwide criticism involved a normal male child, an identical twin born in 1965, whose penis had been damaged during circumcision when a doctor used an electric cauterizing needle instead of a scalpel. The surge of intense heat burned the boy's penis beyond repair and it dried up and sloughed off. The parents, living in a rural community, had no idea of what kind of medical resources were available. They were finally able to get a consultation with a plastic surgeon, who advised them that they could raise their child as a girl. The child had been raised as a boy even though he did not have a penis, but since he had not yet begun to talk, the parents and surgeons felt that he could undergo the reassignment and surgery to make him a girl. They explained that although a phalloplasty surgery could be performed to make an artificial penis with a skin graft, it would have no feeling and would not be able to erect. Further, urination would be subject to leakage and frequent infections (Money and Tucker 1975). When he was 21 months old, he was brought to Johns Hopkins for surgery. At that time, his testicles were removed, a stoma was created for urination, and plastic surgery created flaps from the scrotal skin to look like a vagina. He was renamed Brenda. At four years of age, despite all the attempts of the parents to surround Brenda with dolls, dress like a girl, and be neat and dainty, she preferred to play with her brother's toys. When she entered school, she was not well behaved, and was described as a tomboy. Meanwhile, John Money, the physician who had arranged for the sexual reassignment surgery and psychological counseling, was publishing the results and giving talks about nature versus nurture, the role of hormones in human sexual identity. It is unclear if Money did not know that Brenda was not a completely successful sex reassignment case. Either Dr. Money did not receive negative information, or he ignored the facts, because around the same time that Brenda was supposed to undergo surgery to create an artificial vagina, her parents did not bring her to the hospital. Brenda, after struggling for years with not wanting to be a girl and not knowing why, was finally uninformed about her real sex and the truth about her botched circumcision. She now understood why she felt so different and changed her name to David. David set out to undo what years of socialization, and hormonal and surgical treatment had done, and underwent a double mastectomy. He began a series of testosterone injections and received testicular implants. The male hormones created muscle definition and the implants created a male-appearing scrotum. By this time (1987), plastic surgery was far more sophisticated for rebuilding or creating an artificial penis. Unlike the phalloplasty available when he was seven months old, the new penis was not merely a tube of flaccid tissue. It was constructed with microsurgery in a 12-stage operation that took 13 hours. Three surgeons used the flesh, nerves, and an artery from his right wrist to make a tube for a new urethra and costal cartilage to give support. David would be able to perform sexual intercourse and experience sexual sensation.

David's experience completely contradicted the theory that humans were psychosexually neutral at birth and that, regardless of original genitalia or genotype, with counseling and hormonal treatment, they could be assigned either a male or a female identity. David's case was actually an experiment because previous "sex change" operations had only been performed on adults, individuals such as Christine Jorgenson, a man originally, who had wanted to become a woman. David was different than either an intersex or a transsexual child because he had been born a biologically normal male child. He demonstrated that not all individuals can be socialized to assume an alternative gender role. Fortunately, his transformation never was complete because he often refused to take the hormone pills and refused to have the internal plastic surgery to finish the vaginal canal at puberty. As a teen and later as an adult, David felt that he would have been better off if he had been allowed to maintain his male identity. As an aside, the counseling that was supposed to help him was so upsetting that he eventually refused to attend. If there is any conclusion to this dilemma, it is that "future sex reassignment decisions should be made with maximum sophistication in regard to the implications, psychosocial and psychosexual, of brain development as it is influenced by the intrauterine hormonal milieu. In turn, such brain development influences postnatal psychosexual development" (Reiner 1997, 224).

The Paradox of Congenital Adrenal Hyperplasia

But there is another issue that results from surgery to "normalize" rather than change an individual. A female child was born who appeared to be male because of her enlarged clitoris and fused labia. However, she had ovaries, a uterus, and no testicles. Her parents were told that she had congenital adrenal hyperplasia, and at age 12 she had surgery to reduce the size of her clitoris and to correct her urethra. When her sister was born, she had the same condition, but the clitorectomy became infected and she was left with very little tissue. Both children had to undergo multiple surgeries and endure studies that involved ingesting large quantities of salt, which would make them sick. In conditions where the adrenal glands are involved, salt metabolism is an important function and that is why the experimenters subjected the girls to those studies. They had to undergo repeated examinations and measurements, and as a result, were extremely unhappy. One daughter was angry that her mother had put her through such indignities and exposures. She felt that she was "raped, medically raped" and justifiably felt that way (Feder 2006). Her surgery was extensive because the fused labia had to be separated and her urethra had to be redesigned so that it connected to her vagina. Neither child enjoyed playing with dolls, and both matured to be gay as adults.

On the other hand, a genetically XX individual had lived all his life as a man because he looked like a man. When he developed gynecomastia (breasts), he underwent bilateral mastectomies but the tissue grew back, so he consulted another plastic surgeon. His CAH presented itself as an individual with mixed secondary sexual characteristics. His facial hair showed a male distribution, as did his chest and groin. His muscular pattern was male, but his body fat distribution was female: in the hips, thighs, and breast. His voice was higher than a normal male and lower than an average female. He had a large clitoris and had his one ovary removed surgically. He did not have a uterus. Other than those surgeries, he did not choose to have other modifications, because function was more important to him than appearance.

Support and Information for the Future

An increasing number of intersex individuals are now quite vocal in their comments about their bodies. They create websites with blogs, organizations, and support groups. Although the parents of newborns and hospital personnel are anxious to settle any ambiguous questions regarding sex, this is not necessarily the best decision in all cases. Society, in general, is uncomfortable with an indeterminate category regarding sex, or anything ambiguous about sex that is not defined or understood. The Internet has spawned a huge number of sites where intersex people have a voice, an opportunity that was not possible prior to social media networks. Since there are so many varieties of intersex individuals, there is no single answer for all of them. What research has shown is that parents want to "normalize" their children as much as possible, even if it means sacrificing sexual function. In other words, parents feel that their children will suffer less from ridicule and name calling if they look like other children, that appearance is more important than function. Intersex individuals however, feel that they have been robbed of the opportunity to learn about sexuality, their own kind of sexuality if they were subjected to plastic surgery to modify their genitals before an age when they could give consent. Many of them state that they would rather have put up with stares and comments as children if it meant that sexual function would be preserved.

What Does "Normality" Really Mean?

And then there is the issue of what is the "normal" size for a clitoris. If clitoris size does not interfere with function, why do parents and physicians recommend clitorectomies for girls who have enlarged clitorises? In London, in the mid-18th century, Isaac Baker-Brown, who referred to himself as a British physician, recommended and performed amputations of the clitoris for a variety of "diseases," although he did not differentiate between hyptertrophied and normal-sized clitorises (Baker-Brown 1864). In America, during the early 1940s, Robert Latou Dickinson believed that the size of genitals "offered evidence not only of innate deviance, but also of deviant sexual experiences" (Terry 1995, 141). There was a time period from the mid-19th to the mid-20th century that a medical fad for performing clitorectomies victimized many normal girls and women. At that time, deviance was equated with masturbation, sexual promiscuity, or orgasm. Well-behaved wives and mothers were asexual; to experience pleasure was reason to have the operation performed. Baker-Brown wrote up his many case histories where he allegedly restored women to normal functioning by surgically removing their clitoris.

Changing Sex

Another issue, perhaps where the most publicized about plastic surgery, refers to transsexual adults who choose to change their sex. These are people born with normal genitalia, who felt all their lives that they were men living in women's bodies or women living in men's bodies. Those individuals are referred to as transsexuals (Armstrong 1980, 90). They have made their choices as adults. They undergo body modification surgically and require hormone supplements for the remainder of their lives. In order for them to have the sex-change surgery, they must undergo extensive psychological counseling before, during, and after because the surgery is so drastic and the transition requires many years. The first transsexual to make national headlines was Christine Jorgensen, in 1950 who was originally a male named George. She traveled to Copenhagen to have her surgery and returned to the United States. Then after a hiatus of news regarding this drastic lifestyle change, a male ophthalmologist who became Renee Richards was denied participation in the 1976 U.S. Open Tennis Association because she was not born a female. Both transsexual individuals received extensive media attention.

Not so with Walter Carlos, the musician well known for popularizing Bach and developing the moog synthesizer, who became Wendy Carlos in 1972 when he underwent a sex-change operation. Few people realized that he had made this change. In a *Playboy* interview, he told the writer, "I remember being convinced I was a little girl, not knowing why my parents didn't see it clearly. I didn't understand why they insisted on treating me like a little boy" (Anonymous 1979, 75). Carlos talked about his feelings as a young person: "Transsexuality is a crash course in dealing with the fear of rejection. I was raised as a boy. I wanted love . . . in my head I had this obsession that is among my earliest memories" (104). Now that he has had the surgery, he feels that he has "achieved the removal of one very large negative in [his] life . . . now that he has solved the gender crisis" (100).

One male-to-female transsexual photographer, an activist and member of Transgender Nation, describes her identity this way: "The missing ingredient in most representations of transsexuals is 'the sense of satisfaction we feel about ourselves and our body changes . . . it takes a lot of guts to acknowledge how uncomfortable you are before transition and to willfully accept the challenge of recreating yourself'" (Stryker 1998, 79).

Complexity, Challenges, and Controversy

Any plastic surgery on human genitals is an extremely powerful modification that makes most people uncomfortable because of their beliefs regarding what nature intended. The paradox of ambiguous genitalia is that most parents are unable to deal with the difference and want to change what they see as soon as possible. Yet, many of the grown children who were surgically changed and psychologically reassigned do not agree with what was done to them. They feel mutilated, betrayed, isolated, confused, and angry. David Reimer, the boy who had been raised as Brenda until he was 12, told his biographer, "It just seems that they implied that you're nothing if your penis is gone. The second you lose that, you're nothing, and they've got to do surgery and hormones to turn you into something. Like you're a zero. It's like your whole personality, everything about you is all directed—all pinpointed—toward what's between the legs" (Colapinto 2000, 262). He asks whether if a woman lost her breasts, they would turn her into a man. But even though that's not the same situation, because he's comparing a grown woman to a helpless newborn; the quandary is that society is insistent that gender match biology.

Equally distressed are individuals born with XY chromosomes (i.e., genetically male) whose bodies look female. Many of these young people were surgically altered before they could give their consent. Their internal organs consisted of undescended testicles rather than a uterus and ovaries, and they had a clitoris that was longer than usual. The most traumatizing aspect of the surgery was that they were never told the truth about their bodies. In one case, the girl did not find out the name of her condition until she was 23, 11 years after she had undergone surgery for removal of her testicles and reduction in the size of her clitoris. Other children were less fortunate because the surgery for reduction of clitoral size resulted in complete amputation of the organ (Moreno 1998). This condition, where an individual appears to be female but has neither uterus or ovaries but often has a larger than average clitoris is known as AIS (androgen insensitivity syndrome). It was once called testicular feminization syndrome, and it depends on two conditions that develop while the individual is still a sexually undifferentiated embryo. Initially, all individuals begin with a genital tubercle, urethral fold, and genital swelling (Sadler 1990). If the individual has an XY genetic makeup, during development, one hormone turns on and another turns off, in order to make this individual a male. The first error occurs if, for some reason, that XY individual does not respond the normal secretion of androgen (male hormone), and even though the testicular tissue is present in the embryo, the testes do not develop normally. Therefore, the external genitals remain female-appearing. The second event is not really an error. It is what should happen in a normal male and since the individual is genetically male, the hormones that ordinarily suppress female development (Mullerian inhibitory factor) prevent the ovaries and the uterus from developing. However, since the individual appears to be a female externally, but is really a male genetically, "she" cannot reproduce because she does not have a uterus or ovaries.

Since the early days of John Money's sexual reassignment studies, a great deal of controversy regarding his studies as well as what is the "right" thing to do when an individual's biology does not conform to society's constructs. The problem is so complex that no single answer can apply to every situation. The best that parents can do is to become informed regarding the alternatives and evaluate the ramifications carefully before deciding on any kind of surgery or raising a boy as a girl, or a girl as a boy. In Section III, there is a list of organizations and societies that are specifically dedicated to share information regarding their transsexual, intersex, or nonconventional sexual identity.

REFERENCES

Anonymous. 1979. "Wendy/Walter Carlos." *Playboy* (May): 75–76, 81–86, 91–92, 95–96, 100–4.

Armstrong, C.N. 1980. "Transsexualism: A Medical Perspective." *Journal of Medical Ethics* 6 (2): 90–91.

Baker-Brown, Issac. 1864. *On the Curability of Certain Forms of Insanity, Epilepsy, Catalepsy and Hysteria in Females.* London: Churchill.

Colapinto, John. 2000. *As Nature Made Him.* New York: HarperCollins.

Feder, Ellen, K. 2006. "In Their Best Interests." In *Surgically Shaping Children,* ed. Erik Parens, 189–210. Baltimore: Johns Hopkins University Press.

Hillman, Thea. 2008. *Intersex: For Lack of a Better Word.* San Francisco: Manic D Press.

Money, John. 1968. *Sex Errors of the Body: Dilemmas, Education, Counseling.* Baltimore: Johns Hopkins Press.

Money, John, and Patricia Tucker. 1975. *Sexual Signatures: On Being a Man or a Woman.* Boston: Little Brown.

Moreno, Angela. 1998. "Am I a Woman or a Man?" *Mademoiselle* (March): 178–81, 208.

Paré, Ambröise. 1982. *On Monsters and Marvels,* trans. Janis L. Pallister. Chicago: University of Chicago Press.

Reiner, William. 1997. "To Be Male or Female—That Is the Question." *Archives of Pediatric and Adolescent Medicine* 151 (3): 224–25.

Sadler, T.W. 1990. *Langman's Medical Embryology.* Baltimore: Williams and Wilkins.

Stryker, Susan. 1998. Portrait of a New Man. In *Human Sexuality 98/99,* ed. Susan J. Bunting, 78–79. Guilford, CT: Dushkin/McGraw-Hill.

Terry, Jennifer. 1995. "Anxious Slippages between 'Us' and 'Them': A Brief History of the Scientific Search for Homosexual Bodies." In *Deviant Bodies,* ed. Jennifer Terry and Jacqueline Urla, 110–29. Bloomington: Indiana University Press.

CHAPTER 20

Why Would Anyone Want to Do That?

Television is an interesting medium. The programs that garner the most attention are those that show the human animal in very uncomfortable, often extreme, situations: being subjected to intimate, personal questions by a professional interviewer; undergoing various types of deprivation; competing to see who can lose the most weight; modifying their bodies with piercings, tattoos, and decorations that appear to ablate normal functioning; competitions to torture, embarrass, or "out" hidden truths. Who will survive these rites the most elegantly? Who will allow the entire world to watch a surgical procedure? One might question when the concept of privacy or dignity disappeared. If one has seen *Dr. 90201, Extreme Makeover, Bridal Plasty, The Swan,* or MTV's *Celebrity Look-Alike,* plastic surgery looks like an option at a travel agency, a magical solution to correct any and all face or body imperfections. This chapter will look at some of the issues and controversies that have arisen because of the popularity and appeal of modern plastic surgery with its emphasis on esthetics and perfection.

PLASTIC SURGERY IN YOUR LIVING ROOM

Dr. 90210 is what is referred to as a "reality TV" program because it features actual patients and doctors (rather than actors) who talk about their procedures. In one episode, a married 43-year-old male "virgin" wants to undergo a plastic surgery procedure for a hidden penis because he has been unable to consummate his three-year marriage. He has a number of complicating issues: he is overweight and has an abundance of abdominal fat that virtually covers his penis, a defect in one hip socket, and one leg that is seven inches shorter than the other. The surgeon plans to implant an erection chamber in the patient's penis so that his penis sticks out further and does not appear as hidden under the excessive tissue.

The *Bridalplasty* website informs its readers: "Brides-to-be compete in challenges to earn plastic-surgery procedures in a quest to win their ultimate dream wedding." In small print under BRIDALPLASTY are the words: "the only contest where the winner gets cut." In the first phase of the contest, women who are already engaged complete a series of challenges and fill out a plastic surgery wish list to win a surgery of her choice. Each week, one person is eliminated as the challenges proceed. At the end of the 11 weeks, the remaining bride receives the "wedding of her dreams" and multiple plastic surgeries from her list. Since the show focuses on the glamour and ease with which surgeries are requested and performed, young viewers should be cautioned that plastic surgery is not a trivial matter and the type of perfection that is stressed is unrealistic. This is a TV show and although it is referred to as "reality," most women would not submit to such radical changes to an already perfectly presentable face and body. Marriage is a lifetime commitment; the wedding day is only one out of many. The hostess ends each episode with the dire statement, "Your wedding will still go on, but it will not be perfect" (because no matter how much one plans, there is apt to be something that goes wrong).

The Swan, another reality TV show, ran for two years from 2004 until 2006. Its name referred to the Hans Christian Anderson story about the ugly duckling who became a beautiful swan when he grew up. For the show, patients who considered themselves ugly were chosen to undergo beautifying procedures, often a combination of plastic surgery, orthodontics, and maxillofacial surgery. Each week, two contestants would be presented, but only one would be chosen for the procedures and prizes. Their blurb is, "Do you have a dream that you haven't achieved because of how you look? Do you believe that if you got the looks you always wanted, you could then go on to achieve your deepest desires—including winning a beauty pageant? If so, producers of *The Swan* might be interested in hearing from you" (*The Swan* n.d.).

Extreme Makeover ran from 2002 to 2007. The contestants for this program had to audition and if chosen were awarded plastic surgery, dental and orthodontic treatment, hairstyling, and wardrobe advice. But despite its fairy godmother promises and dramatic makeovers that were seen by viewers, not everyone benefited. One woman with a pronounced overbite, stringy hair, and small breasts was scheduled for eyelid surgery, an otoplasty (ear surgery), implants, dental surgery, and maxillofacial surgery. In order to emphasize her ugliness and "before" status, the family was interviewed and asked to describe her. This was a routine procedure for the producers because it made the results after the surgery all the more impressive. However, when the producers realized that all those changes could not be accomplished in their designated time slot, they dropped the patient without warning. When the formerly eager contestant returned home as "Cinderella" rather than as a dazzling princess, she was emotionally traumatized, particularly because of the previous comments made by her close relatives. Four months later, her sister, who had been quite vocal regarding the contestant's ugliness, committed suicide, allegedly from guilt feelings. The rejected contestant sued *ABC*, blaming them for her sister's suicide, and settled for an amount unknown.

ALTERED IDENTITIES

As if those programs were not sufficient to illustrate how bizarre one could get with plastic surgery, to escalate the interest one more notch, a program on MTV called *I Want a Famous Face* interviews individuals, most young adults, who intentionally changed their appearance, not to look better or to rid themselves of an ugly feature but to totally alter their appearance, lose their identity, and look exactly like a favorite celebrity. Twelve people chose to have these remakes and then appear on MTV to be interviewed. The first, Gia, who describes herself as a "26-year-old transsexual porn star turned director/producer" wants to look like the actress, Pamela Anderson. She has had breast implants, liposuction on her abdomen and chin, a rhinoplasty, micrografts to her hairline, and fat transferred to her smile lines. Two of her surgeries, the breast implants and the rhinoplasty, were done a second time. One might question a number of her motives. First of all, even if the surgery to change from male to female or vice versa were regarded as usual, why would someone want to look like another person? In this case, could this pattern of multiple surgeries reflect a BDD to begin with and a condition referred to as polysurgery, where the patient continues to seek surgeries to solve emotional problems? Since the interviewer does not delve into these personal areas, the viewers are left uninformed regarding Gia's possible psychological needs.

"Nikicia" wanted to look like Janet Jackson. Her plastic surgeries were designed to make her body thinner so that she can market herself as an actress/singer. How ironic that the sister of the child star *cum* "thriller" singer who had more than 22 plastic surgery procedures to change his looks would be a model for someone else. Perhaps this illustrates the maxim about beauty being in the eye of the beholder, or the French maxim, *chacun á son gout* (each to his own taste).

"Audrey" was an aspiring model who wanted to look like Jessica Simpson. She decided that her small breasts need to be augmented with implants because they were keeping her from "reaching the big time." This is an example of a patient who has focused on a body part and is blaming it rather than anything else about herself (e.g., her face, height, weight, education, speech, hairstyle) as a reason that she does not have the career she wants. What will happen to her if she does get implants and she does not become a big time model? Will she try to look like another actress? Or will she finally accept reality?

If there could be one more symptom of a person who used plastic surgery for an unusual goal, it was the woman wanted to look like Barbie, the 11.5"-tall Mattel doll that was popular during the 1960s (Kershaw 2002). Barbie was the subject of a great many feminist critiques because she had an abnormal, unnatural body (Leung 2004). Unlike most dolls, she was not a baby, she was a pre-teen creation. Her chest was 4.3", her waist 3.5", and her hips 5". Her shoulder-length blond hair was just wavy enough to not be straight and her eyes were blue. When researchers estimated how she would look as a 5"6" woman, they came up with the dimensions 39, 21, 33 (which do not explain the proportionally smaller hip measurement). The first person who wanted to have plastic surgery to look like Barbie was Cindy Jackson, a 23-year-old American who did not consider herself attractive. She underwent a series of 31 surgeries over a period of 14 years. She had two rhinoplasties; laser surgery on her forehead, upper eyes and lower eyes; cheek implants; four facelifts; a chin reduction; chemicals peels; and surgery to shorten the gap between her nose and her mouth. She had eyebrows, eyeliner, lip liner, and lipstick tattooed onto her face. The second woman to undergo multiple surgeries to look like Barbie was a 49-year-old British citizen, a former Playboy Bunny. Sarah Burge spent 539,500 pounds (close to $600,000 at the time) for 100 plastic surgery procedures to make herself look like Barbie (Rutherford 2010). Sarah might have had a different original motivation to begin her series of surgeries. Unlike Cindy, she had facial reconstructive surgery after being beaten up and left for dead. In an article online, she poses a paradox. Regarding plastic surgery, she states "It's addictive—you find yourself wondering what you can have done next?" but then goes on to say: "It's not that I'm unhappy with the way I look—I've always been confident about my appearance." There is an obvious disconnect here. She states: "That's why I want to keep my body and face as they are. All the work I've had done has been to stop the ageing process." But all one needs to do is look at her before and after pictures to see that she did not keep her body and face as they were. And, of course, she will not be able to stop the ageing process, only certain outward aspects of it.

MEDICAL TOURISM

These extreme examples represent what the media moguls think is important to present to the public about plastic surgery. In contrast to the invasive and hyperbolic nature of TV programs, if one desires privacy, the best way to obtain that is to actually travel to a place where no one will know the patient. This is accomplished now by an entirely different type of travel, referred to as cosmetic surgery tourism, a package deal where the patient buys airfare to South Africa, Brazil, Jamaica, Bolivia, Mexico, Costa Rica, Venezuela, Thailand, or other venues. One advertisement from a company called Cosmetic Surgery Travel includes testimonials from former patients. They include Dianna, who wrote:

> I had a breast augmentation procedure in Bangkok . . . arranged by Cosmetic Surgery Travel. My husband and I are very, very happy with the results of the surgery and the whole experience. Thank you . . . for organizing everything so well and so professionally. I highly recommend Cosmetic Surgery Travel to anyone who is considering breast implants or any other plastic surgery. The hospital was the best and the staff was great. And of course, my doctor was perfect! The best thing was the cost. I saved a couple thousand dollars and the cost was exactly what you said it would be.

And Lizzie:

> I'm having WOW moments with my new figure and feel great. Just stopped wearing the compression girdle today. It's fun to know that I will even get smaller as the swelling goes down, but the numbness is pretty much gone. I still can't believe how good my recovery was. I have spread the word about your services and given out your website. Thanks again for everything.

One website from Brazil gives a figure of 48,000 patients who sought plastic surgery in 2005 (Heelan 2005).

Cultural Relativity

It appears that there is no limit to what lengths people will go to obtain a surgical procedure. Likewise, the body parts remaining that have not been modified in some way are very few. Western industrialized cultures are outraged and abhor the practice referred to as female genital mutilation, where Muslim and other cultures in Africa amputate the clitoris of little girls at the age of 6 or 7. Yet in the Western culture, they make choices to reduce the size of a female child's clitoris if it happens to look "too large" or modify a boy's genitals routinely by circumcision. Since this is a body part not exhibited daily, it does seem strange that so much attention should be paid to its appearance instead of function. Unfortunately, one unintended result of surgery on ambiguous genitalia is that the individual could be denied sexual sensation if the surgery is not performed correctly. The question contrasts the attitude and viewpoint of the parent versus the result that will affect the child for the rest of his or her life. The parent is concerned with how the child will compare with other children. But the grown child might resent that a choice was made which is now socially crippling. Two such cases were discussed in detail in Chapter 19.

Despite Western culture's label of female genital mutilation referring to the "other," a series of female genital procedures have been popularized in the United States referred to as "vaginal rejuvenation" and or "designer vaginas." It is unclear if physicians began to market this to women or if women requested that doctors perform these procedures, but an array of procedures do exist and evidently are ubiquitous enough to be a standard package offered on many websites. One website (Matlock n.d.) states that the doctors have trained 250 surgeons in 43 countries to perform female genital plastic surgery. The terminologies that they have trademarked are "Laser Vaginal Rejuvenation®, and Designer Laser Vaginoplasty®. Laser Vaginal Rejuvenation is a procedure that tightens the vagina for the "enhancement of sexual gratification." It does not say for whose gratification. Designer Laser Vaginoplasty (DLV) is for "the aesthetic enhancement of vulvar structures," otherwise known as labioplasty or labiaplasty. Another doctor refers to labiaplasty as "labia reduction and beautification" (Stern 2011). This website states that at one time, labiaplasties were only performed on entertainers, models, or performers, but today, the "importance of female genitalia are much more prevalent" (Stern 2011). The doctor goes on to say that large labia "may cause severe embarrassment with a sexual partner or a loss in self-esteem," not to mention pain and discomfort. He states that there are both medical and aesthetic reasons for the surgery. The medical reasons are that overly large lips can cause discomfort or irritation because of the friction from tight pants that one wears during exercise. Vaginoplasty is not new. It is a procedure that has been done at least for 40 years for women when traumatic childbearing caused damages to the pelvic floor, often resulting in urinary leakage. But what is new is the way it is being marketed. The website states that "many women with grown children are now seeking renewal of the vaginal tissues-vaginal tightening-specifically to enhance the sexual experience they have with loving mates" (Stern 2011, 3). The aesthetic reasons are less explicit. Those reasons include "being driven by societal evolution regarding sexual habits, wants and expectations." Exactly what the doctor means by societal evolution is not at all clear, but from an anthropological standpoint, sexual behaviors in humans have probably never changed: only the disclosure regarding the practices has. And mass media, particularly the Internet, has facilitated that aspect of learning about sexual behaviors. He goes on to say that, "most women seek sculpting of the labia or vaginal beautification to achieve a better look for themselves and their sexual partner." As a result of this ad, will women begin to look at their labia more often?

As an aside, the African group of people referred to as Hottentots (now referred to as the Khoisan), during the 19th century, would pull and stretch the labia of their female children from the earliest years, making an apron that sometimes extended to the mid-thigh or lower. They believed this cultural practice made their women more beautiful and marriageable: the epitome of pulchritude was to have long external labia that flapped when one walked. Perhaps this confirms the plasticity of human attitudes as well as the body.

REFERENCES

Heelan, Charis Atlas. 2005. "Cosmetic Surgery Tourism: A Tummy Tuck in Thailand, a Breast Augmentation in Brazil." http://www.frommers.com/articles/3049.

Kershaw, Sarah. 2002. "Ruth Handler, Whose Barbie Gave Dolls Curves, Dies at 85." *New York Times,* April 29.

Leung, Rebecca. 2004. "Becoming Barbie: Living Dolls: Real Life Couple Are Models of Plastic Perfection." http://www.cbsnews.com/ stories/2004/07/29/48hours/main632909.shtml.

Matlock, David. n.d. "About Dr. Matlock." http://www.drmatlock.com/Meet DrMatlock.html.

Rutherford, Nick. 2010. "Pictured: The Forty-something ex-Bunny Girl Who Has Spent Half a Million Pounds Having 100 Cosmetic Surgery Operations to Turn Herself into a Real-life Barbie." August 9. http://www.dailymail.co.uk/femail/article-1080930/Pictured-The-ex-Bunny-Girl-whos-spent-half-million-pounds-turn-real-life-Barbie.html.

Stern, Bernard. 2011. Labiaplasty.com Discreet and Confidential help for women. http://www.labiaplastysurgeon.com/dr-stern-testimonials.html.

The Swan. www.realitytvworld.com/news/fox-seeking-female-ugly-ducklings-for-new-the-swan-reality-makeover-series-1847.php.

Section III

Introduction

In addition to the interesting history of plastic surgery from wartime to supermodel, the reader must be aware of information produced by the accepted medical authorities regarding various procedures and practices. Because of the availability of too much information in magazines, on entertainment television shows, and on the Internet, the publishers of this series feel it is in the public interest for potential patients to learn factual information about plastic surgery. These primary documents are the result of research, often government research on controversial issues or questions that surfaced after a number of patients sought medical advice.

This information includes the 2006 FDA New Release about silicone breast implants, a glossary, a timeline, some information about intersex and transsexual individuals, and the ethical organizations and societies that provide training to doctors and publications to patients. There is also an additional bibliography of reading material, some more technical than the level of this book for those interested in researching some of these topics.

Documents

1: CASES OF DEFORMITY FROM BURNS, SUCCESSFULLY TREATED BY PLASTIC OPERATIONS, THOMAS MÜTTER, 1843

Thomas Dent Mütter (1811–1859) was a surgeon with an extensive collection of pathological specimens, wax models, and surgical instruments he had collected during his lifetime. In 1858 he donated his collection to the College of Physicians of Philadelphia so that medical students and other doctors could benefit from the educational value and have the opportunity to conduct research using those unusual, interesting, and historical articles. Among his specialties were club foot, cleft palate, congenital anomalies, and treatment of burns. He was a plastic surgery pioneer who is best known for the cervical flap that he developed. His special interest was in restoring function to burn victims.

Source: Mütter, Thomas D. *Cases of Deformity from Burns, Successfully Treated by Plastic Operations.* Philadelphia: Merrihew & Thompson, 1843. Reprinted with permission from the Mütter Museum and The College of Physicians of Philadelphia.

Note

Two years and more have elapsed since the first of the operations reported was performed, and the patient still continues relieved. No contraction has taken place, and the success of the experiment may therefore be considered complete; the other cases are also doing well. I have performed similar operations in four other cases since this report was published in the *American Journal of Medical Sciences* for July, 1842, and, with but one exception, complete success has followed in every instance. May 20, 1843.

Cases of Deformity from Burns, Relieved by Operation

In the month of January, 1841, I was requested to attend the Miss A.T. of Chesterfield Township, New Jersey, who for twenty-three years had endured much mental as well as physical inconvenience from the effects of a burn which occurred when she was five years old, and involved the face, throat, and upper part of the thorax in front. The following extract from her history of the case, will explain the nature of the accident, as well as the treatment to which she had been subjected before I saw her:—"I received a burn when five years old by my clothes taking fire. My grandmother, being a great doctress nursed me, until prevented by indisposition; and as they wished me to remain in as comfortable a position as possible, my life began entirely despaired of by the family, medical aid was not called in. Doctor Burns, a neighboring physician, hearing of the circumstances, could not refrain from coming to see me; he called twice as a friend, and was then forbidden to come again until sent for, which was never done. When about 11 years of age, an attempt was made by Dr. Cook, of Bordentown, to afford some relief. Being young, I was much alarmed and opposed him. My near relations, being unwilling to see me suffer, united with me; and he was obliged to desist before completing his design. I therefore did not experience any relief, and have been unable to throw my head to the left side, or backwards, or to close my mouth for more than a few seconds at a time for 23 years. My right eye was also drawn down some distance below the other, and when I endeavored to turn my head, it was entirely closed. My condition has been most humiliating, and made life a burden; but having good health, I strove to reconcile myself to my hard lot!" In addition to the symptoms so vividly described, I found the angles of the lower jaw altered, and the incisor teeth nearly horizontal, (as is seen in cases of chronic hypertrophy of the tongue,) by the pressure of the tongue, which organ, in consequence of the inability of the patient to close the mouth, was always visible, and indeed *protruded,* when she was silent. The clavicle on the right side was also so completely embedded in the cicatrix, that it could scarcely be felt, and there was no external indication of its location. The chin, from the shortness of the bands, was drawn down to within *one inch and a half* of the top of the sternum, and the head consequently inclined very much. The space between the chin and sternum was also filled up by the cicatrix, so that no depression existed in front of her neck. Fig. 1, which represents her full face, affects a very correct idea of her appearance. After carefully examining the case, and fully explaining to the patient and her friends the inability of any of the usual operations for such deformities, I proposed to them one entirely different in its principle, which although severe, as well as somewhat hazardous, promised partial, if not entire relief. To this my patient readily assented, declaring that death was preferable to a

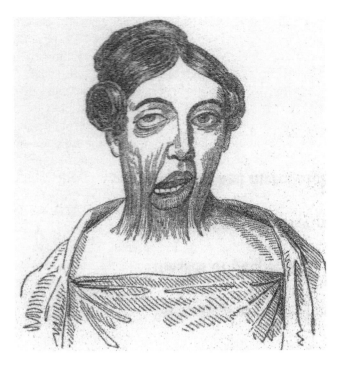

Figure 1. Mütter, Thomas D. *Cases of Deformity from Burns, Successfully Treated by Plastic Operations.* Philadelphia: Merrihew & Thompson, 1843. Reprinted with permission from the Mütter Museum and The College of Physicians of Philadelphia.

life of such misery as hers. In conformity with her wishes, I at once placed her on a preparatory treatment, and on the 12th of January, performed the operation to be described, assisted by Drs. Noble and pierce, and in the presence of Messrs. Ward, Ducachet, Mason and Egan, medical students.

The patient being placed in a strong light, and seated on a low chair, her head was thrown back as far as possible, and sustained in this position by an assistant.

Seating myself in front, I began the operation by making an incision which commenced on the outside of the cicatrix in *sound skin* and passed across the throat into *sound skin* on the opposite side. This penetrated merely through the integuments, and was made as near the centre of the cicatrix as possible. It was therefore about three quarters of an inch above the top of the sternum, and of course in the most vital part of the neck. My object in making it so low down was to get at the attachments of the sterno-cleido-mastoid muscles, which in consequence of the long flexion of the head, were not more than three inches in length, and required on one side *complete*, and on the other *partial* division, before the head could be raised. The integuments having been thus divided, I next carefully dissected through the cicatrix until I reached the fascia superficialis colli, which I could readily detect, and then going on still deeper, I exposed the sterno-cleido-mastoid muscle of the right side, and passing a director under it, as low down as possible, divided both its attachments. This enable me to raise the head an inch or two; but finding that it was still kept down by the sterno-cleido-mastoid of the *left* side, I divided the sternal attachment of this muscle, and was much gratified to find that the head could at once be placed in its proper position, the clavicular attachment of the muscle offering little or no resistance. A most shocking wound, *six inches in length six inches by five* and a half in width, was then made, and yet there was scarcely any hemorrhage ; three of four vessels only requiring the ligature. (See fig. 2.)

The next stop in the operation consisted in the detachment of a flap of *sound skin* with which this chasm could be filled; for I knew very well that if permitted to heal by granulation only, the patient, so far from being benefited, would be made worse than before. To obtain this flap, I commenced at the terminal extremity of the first incision, and carrying the scalpel *downwards and outwards* over the deltoid muscle, dissected up an oval piece of integument *six inches and a half* in *length,* by *six in width,*

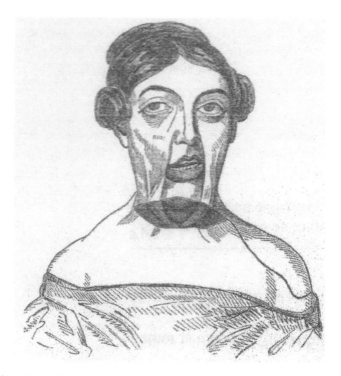

Figure 2. Mütter, Thomas D. *Cases of Deformity from Burns, Successfully Treated by Plastic Operations.* Philadelphia: Merrihew & Thompson, 1843. Reprinted with permission from the Mütter Museum and The College of Physicians of Philadelphia.

leaving it attached at the upper part of the neck, see fig. 2.) This dissection was painful, but not bloody, only one small vessel being opened. The flap thus detached was next brought round by making a half-turn in its pedicle, placed in the gap it was destined to fill, and carefully attached by several twisted sutures, to the edges of the wound. (see fig. 3.)

Several straps were then applied to support the sutures, but no other dressing was deemed as visible. The edges of the wound on the shoulder from which the flap had been removed, were next brought together by straps and sutures, and, with the exception of the upper third, was completely covered in. A pledget of lint moistened with warm water was laid upon the raw surface, a bandage applied by this position, by which the head was carried backwards and the patient put to the bed. The fortitude with which this truly severe operation was borne excited the admiration of all present. Scarcely a groan escaped the patient nor was it necessary to give her a mouthful of wine and water during this whole period of duration.

Rest and quietude were enjoined, and the patient prohibited from taking any kind of nourishment, in order that adhesion or union by the first intention might be accomplished.

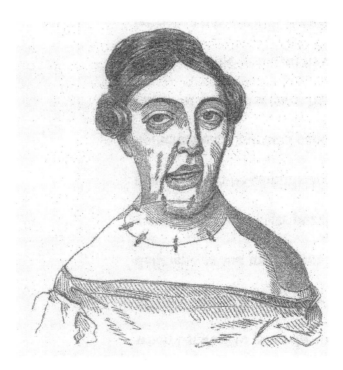

Figure 3.   Mütter, Thomas D. *Cases of Deformity from Burns, Successfully Treated by Plastic Operations*. Philadelphia: Merrihew & Thompson, 1843. Reprinted with permission from the Mütter Museum and The College of Physicians of Philadelphia.

Kam/13th.—Patient has passed a good night; slight acceleration of the pulse, but no fever; not much thirst; complains of *stiffness* in the neck, and pain in the back from lying in one position so long. Slight headache from the anodyne which it was deemed advisable to administer *before* the operation.

14th.—Much as yesterday; a little nervous, but no fever; no swelling or pain in the wound; some thirst and hunger, but willing to go another day without sustenance.

15th.—A little feverish; wound painful at one point, thirst intense, bowels not opened; restless, and anxious; ordered an enema to be administered at once; and spoonfuls of cool barley water to be taken every hour or two.

16th.—Much better; enema operated well, fever gone; thirst less, skin moist; cheerful and in hope.

17th.—The same; took off straps and found the wound united along the edges, with the exception of here and there a point; a small pouch of pus at the most dependent part of the flap; patient rather restless under the dressing.

Evacuated the pus through a small opening in its vicinity; took out some of the pins, reapplied the straps; dressed the shoulder with poultice of slippery elm; ordered a little mutton broth, and an enema of salt and water.

It would be worse than needless to detail the daily symptoms and tx from this time to the period at which the patient was enabled to move about, and enjoy the full benefit of the operation.

It will be sufficient to state that no unfavourable symptom made its appearance, that union by the *first intention* took place throughout the entire wound, with the exception of one small point which united by granulation; that the wound in the shoulder, except just over the acromion process, healed kindly: and that the patient, as her own words will testify has been relieved of all or nearly all inconveniences. The following extract is from a letter received some time since.

"The comfort and satisfaction I feel, cannot be expressed; your exertions in my behalf have been blessed far beyond my most sanguine expectations. You have set my head at liberty, so that I can turn it any way, at pleasure and without pain; you have relieved the drawing of my eye; and I am also able to close my mouth with comfort that cannot be described! "In order to accomplish the closure of my mouth, the lower incisor teeth were straightened, and one of them extracted by a dentist. The angles of the lower jaw have, in consequence of the condition of the throat, regained in a great measure their proper shape, and the whole appearance of the patient is so much altered that persons who saw her before the operation, scarcely recognized her as the same individual. I should have mentioned that one of the troublesome circumstances occurred which will serve as a lesson in all subsequent operations of a similar character. Although very careful to extend my incisions from beyond what I suppose was the extent of the cicatrix, I yet left a band of this tissue, certainly not thicker nor wider than a

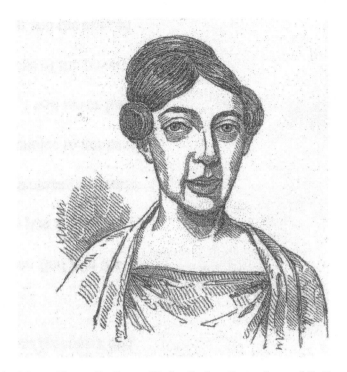

Figure 4.   Mütter, Thomas D. *Cases of Deformity from Burns, Successfully Treated by Plastic Operations*. Philadelphia: Merrihew & Thompson, 1843. Reprinted with permission from the Mütter Museum and The College of Physicians of Philadelphia.

small wire. This band contracted, and before the patient could be entirely relieved, I was obliged to loosen it, by making an incision in the sound skin below on the neck. To support the neck after the incision had healed, I gave this patient a *stiff stock* on which her chin rested, and this instrument also served to press the integuments back, by which the natural excavation or depth of the skin in the front was readily effected. This stock is of course, no longer in use, and the motions of the head are perfect; altho' it was predicted that the antagonism between the muscles on the front and back of the neck, having been in a great degree destroyed by the section of the mastoids, these motions would necessarily never be required. (Fig. 4. Represents her as cured.)

More than a twelvemonth has elapsed since the operation was performed, and yet there is no contraction in the flap, and the relief of the patient is complete.

2: *SAFETY OF SILICONE BREAST IMPLANTS,* 1999

The following is an abstracted executive summary written by the editors for the committee on the Safety of Silicone Breast Implants, Institute of

Medicine, and National Academy of Medicine after public concern. The entire executive summary and the report are available to read online at http://www.nap.edu/catalog/9602.html.

The authors of this document state that the *Safety of Silicone Breast Implants* provides a comprehensive, well-organized review of the science behind one of the most significant medical controversies of our time.

Source: Bondurant, Stuart, Virginia Ernster, and Roger Herdman, eds. *Safety of Silicone Breast Implants.* Washington: National Academy Press, 1999: IX–XI, 1–11. Reprinted with permission by the National Academy of Sciences, Courtesy of the National Academies Press, Washington, D.C.

Preface

To begin, we reflect that the need for this report and the oft-cited deficiencies of the research relevant to silicone breast implants both derive from the fact that silicone breast implants were widely used before there was any requirement for premarket assessment of toxicity and complications or any form of prior approval or licensing for all medical devices. For many years there were no requirements to document the composition of implants or the specific model that was implanted in a particular individual. Further, there was no systematic, comprehensive, postmarketing surveillance of the long-term positive and negative consequences of silicone breast implantation. In the absence of structured requirements for risk assessment before 1992, much of the literature on aspects of silicone breast implants is anecdotal, lacking in appropriate controls, or otherwise of little value in establishing risk. This report stands as strong evidence of the need for thorough and systematic assessment of medical devices prior to their utilization and for continuing assessment after widespread utilization to discover any rare complications that premarketing studies of feasible size might not demonstrate. In the judgment of the committee, however, there have now been sufficient studies of quality to reach a number of well-based conclusions.

Several important events have occurred since this study was initiated. A major class action litigation, brought on behalf of women with silicone breast implants, was settled with a substantial award to the plaintiffs. Meanwhile, a court turned to a panel of experts for advice on specific issues before the court concerning health consequences of silicone breast implants. The report of the National Science Panel . . . is a substantial work that sets forth clearly and definitively the strong scientific evidence not always available in the past to courts with jurisdiction over breast implant litigation. The report of the National Science Panel is a model of the provision to the courts of the best available scientific advice in a matter in which balanced and informed scientific information and judgment are essential. The committee considered whether various known disease-related conditions occur more frequently in women with silicone breast implants than in women in the general population and also whether there might be a novel disease syndrome or syndromes in women with silicone breast implants. To date, proposals for the latter possibility have been based on criteria that are inadequate for scientific evaluation or confirmation. The proposed syndromes often involve ill-defined subjective symptoms that occur with substantial frequency in the general population. Absent a marker or set of markers to confer specificity, the existence of such a syndrome cannot be proven or used to exclude or include any individual or group.

The committee heard directly and indirectly from many women who suffer severe systemic illnesses that they firmly believe are due to their silicone breast implants. Many of these women are seriously ill, and the committee was moved by their suffering. However, the committee is convinced that in most instances the silicone breast implants are not causally related to these illnesses since such illnesses appear to occur at about the same frequency in women with silicone breast implants and in women without implants. On the other hand, the committee was impressed by what appear to be the relatively high frequencies of local complications (such as rupture and contracture) that are unique to women with silicone breast implants. Although they are not life-threatening, these local complications may result in discomfort, inconvenience, disfigurement, pain, and other morbidity and when further corrective procedures are necessary, an additional expense.

Many women with silicone breast implants feel strongly that they were not provided with adequate information as a basis for consenting to have these implants. The committee is aware that recall by patients of the specific conditions and terms of medical consent is imperfect, and it is aware that several medical organizations have worked diligently to improve the quality of informed consent of patients with silicone breast implants. The committee believes, however, that more consistent and higher quality informed consent is possible and, among its recommendations, urges the development and testing of model processes and systems for ensuring fully informed consent for future recipients of silicone breast implants. A successful system may be applicable to other implantable devices in the future.

Executive Summary

In House Report 104–659, which accompanied a 1997 appropriations bill, Congress asked the U.S. Department of Health and Human Services (DHHS) to sponsor a study of the safety of silicone breast implants by the

Institute of Medicine (IOM) of the National Academy of Sciences. Funds were committed from several sources in DHHS, and the National Institute of Arthritis and Musculoskeletal and Skin Diseases (NIAMS) was designated as the lead agency. In late 1997, the IOM agreed to carry out a comprehensive evaluation of the evidence for the association of silicone breast implants, both gel and saline filled, with human health conditions, assemble a comprehensive list of scientific references on this subject, and to consider recommendations for further research. . .

Data and evidence for an association or for no association of a health condition with breast implants were ranked as either conclusive/convincing, limited/suggestive, insufficient, flawed or lacking. A finding of insufficient or absent data was not meant to imply that more information was needed. When this was desirable, and only then, the committee so noted. . . .

Satisfaction is important, both inherently and because women's tolerance for complications influences their demand for medical and surgical interventions to correct implant problems, which in turn has safety implications. Yet surveys of satisfaction are often administered by plastic surgeons, which may bias results and influence women's reporting, and surveys are also often carried out before the likely appearance of some complications. The response rate itself may be influenced by the degree of satisfaction or other personal considerations.

The committee arrived at an estimate of 1.5 million to 1.8 million U.S. women with breast implants in 1997, the year the IOM study began. The committee estimates that about 70% of these implants were performed for augmentation, (i.e., enlarging or changing the appearance of the breast), and 30% for reconstruction, (i.e., restoring the form of the breast after mastectomy for cancer, fibrocystic disease, or other indications). The committee also noted that more than 10 million persons in the United States have some type of implant, such as finger joints or pacemakers, and many of these implants are made, at least in part, from silicone. A short review of regulation by the Food and Drug Administration (FDA) explains why current breast implantation is primarily with saline-filled implants, and describes the effects of government actions on gel-filled, polyurethanecoated, and other implants and on the companies that manufactured them.

Silicon is a semimetallic element, and silicone is a family of silicon-based organic compounds, of which the poly(dimethylsiloxanes) (PDMS) are prominent members. PDMS compounds are polymers, and the length and cross-linking of the polymer chain(s) affect the physical properties of these substances. Implant shells are made from an elastomer, that is, a high molecular weight, cross-linked rubbery substance, and they are filled with silicone gel, a less cross-linked spongy substance permeated with lower molecular weight silicone fluids. Other fillers are possible and include primarily saline.

. . . . The committee was struck by the great number of changes in silicone breast implants since they were introduced in 1962. These changes have created different "generations" of gel-filled implants, which may have very different effects. The changes were introduced with little or no pretesting for biological or clinical effects as far as the committee could determine. Varying control of the diffusion of silicone fluid through gel implant shells, shell strength, and therefore durability of both gel- and saline-filled implants, and polyurethane coating were among the changes that affected the clinical performance of silicone breast implants in ways that were not predicted in many instances. The history and implications of polyurethane coating of breast implants were reviewed, although polyurethane implants have not been available from U.S. manufacturers since 1991. On the other hand, changes have been made that have improved implants, as plastic surgeons and manufacturers have learned from reports of problems with existing implant models. Barrier shells, texturing, better valves in saline implants, and stronger shells that are more resistant to rupture or deflation have been some of these changes.

Study of the toxicology of silicones began in the 1940s. Although these studies were consistent with the standards of the day, in hindsight they fall short of current regulatory requirements; in particular, more chronic, long-term studies would have been desirable. As would be expected for any large family of organic compounds, some silicones have toxic or biologic effects, but PDMS fluids, gels, and elastomers were generally well tolerated on injection or implantation. Like other polymers, silicone can induce "solid state" carcinogenesis in rodents, but there is no evidence that this occurs in humans. Studies of the reproductive toxicology of PDMS have been negative. Several studies of the distribution of silicones from depots of experimental gel implantation or fluid injection have shown that silicones remain localized where deposited and that low molecular weight silicones which may be mobile to a small extent, are cleared from the body after relatively short half-lives. Since the evidence is lacking or flawed that amorphous silica in breast implant shells is available to, or found in tissues of experimental animals or humans, or that crystalline silica is formed or present at any time in women with implants, the toxicology of silica has not been reviewed, although literature on silica is included in the references. Some investigators have asserted that platinum catalysts in breast implants may diffuse through the implant shell, be present in multivalent states, and provoke toxic reactions. The evidence currently available suggests that platinum is present only in the zero valence elemental state. Evidence does not suggest there are high concentrations in implants, significant diffusion of platinum out of implants, or platinum toxicity in humans. In general, the committee has concluded that a review of the toxicology studies of silicones known to be used in breast implants does not provide a basis for concern at expected exposures.

. . . . The committee considered local complications an important aspect of the story of breast implantation—historically, now, and in the future—for women considering these implants.

. . . . In general, the committee concludes that complications are frequent. Specific complications discussed include implant rupture and deflation, contracture of the fibrous tissue capsule around implants, and elevated silicone concentrations in peri-implant tissues. Results with saline versus gel implants, barrier implants, textured implants, steroid-treated implants and implants in different positions are discussed. The infections, hematomas, and pain that may accompany implants are also considered. A number of factors affect the integrity of the silicone elastomer implant shell. These include: shell thickness and strength which can vary considerably; untoward events such as needle sticks and other trauma associated with the vagaries of daily life, including closed capsulotomies, which the committee concludes should be abandoned; and the abrasion and wear of the implant shell in the body enhanced by wrinkling and fold flaws. Precise frequencies of the rupture of gel-filled, or the deflation of saline-filled, implants are not available. The properties of these devices that can affect rupture or deflation have changed markedly over time, and particularly in the case of gel implants, it has not been possible to reliably diagnose and study rupture in an unbiased cross section of implanted women. It is safe to say however that, like any device, breast implants have a finite life span. Rupture frequencies, in the past, have been considerable, and the rupture rate of current models has yet to be measured over the relevant periods of time. The deflation of saline implants is more easily diagnosed, but 100% discovery of deflations does not occur, and deflation frequencies of current models remain to be measured reliably.

Breast implants, like any foreign body, incite a surrounding fibrous tissue reaction. This fibrous capsule may contract, distorting the appearance of the implanted breast and causing pain. Contracture may be apparent as early as a few months after implantation, and the committee finds that it most likely continues over prolonged periods of time. As with any biologic reaction, some variation in contracture may be expected. The severity of contracture can differ in the breasts of the same woman. The exact frequency of contracture is not known because it has varied from 100% with pre-silicone implants to much lower prevalences, depending on a number of factors, as modern silicone implants have evolved. Few studies that have measured contracture have controlled all except one study variable.

Silicon or silicone levels are elevated in capsular and sometimes breast tissue around implants, and this may contribute to capsular contracture. The committee has found suggestive evidence that contracture frequency is lessened by saline implants and barrier shells that, among other things, diminish the exposure of peri-implant breast tissue to silicone. Construction of an implant shell with projections, known as texturing, also appears to control contracture. The committee reviewed the evidence on the effects of adrenal corticosteroids on capsular contracture. Although some data suggest that they may reduce contractures, steroids also cause damage to surrounding breast tissue, are not an FDA approved or manufacturer-recommended usage, and may weaken elastomer implant shells. A number of studies have shown that bacteria can be cultured from normal breast tissue, even at some depth below the surface of the skin. These bacteria are skin flora that reside in the lactiferous ducts of the normal breast, and often can be cultured from implants, where they may contribute from time to time to infections. There is suggestive evidence that the presence of bacteria correlates with contracture. A few investigators have reported finding an association between the presence of bacteria around implants and systemic symptoms or breast pain, although this evidence is limited. Hematomas, or collections of blood around implants, have also been proposed as causes of contracture. Evidence for this is insufficient. Significant contractures are reported considerably more frequently than clinically observable hematomas. Pain is also a problem in some women with implants. A number of studies report pain that has resulted in considerable discomfort and led to the removal of implants. The committee reached three major general conclusions regarding local and perioperative complications. First, these complications occur frequently enough to be a cause for concern and to justify the conclusion that they are the primary safety issue with silicone breast implants. Among others, these include overall reoperations, ruptures or deflations, contractures, infections, hematomas, and pain. Second, risks accumulate over the lifetime of the implant, but quantitative data on this point are lacking for modern implants and are deficient historically for a number of reasons that have been noted in this report. Among these are lack of data from representative samples of the population, lack of information on implant characteristics that affect complications, and lack of precise and reliable detection of complications. Third, information concerning the nature and relatively high frequency of local complications and reoperations is an essential element of adequate informed consent for women undergoing breast implantation.

Chapters 6 through 8 evaluate the immunology of silicone, the relationship of antinuclear and other autoantibodies to breast implants, and the association of breast implants with classic connective tissue disease, undifferentiated connective tissue disease, and proposed new signs, symptoms, or novel disease. Studies in experimental animals have reported modest adjuvant effects of silicone gel and some silicone fluids, but no clinical implications of adjuvant effects have been discovered. Human adjuvant disease is not a defined disease, and the term should be abandoned. Other animal studies have not elucidated a role for silicone in immune disease. Cytokine assays have not provided conclusive evidence of immune activation. Evidence for silicone as a superantigen is insufficient. Modest decreases in natural killer cell activity have been reported after exposure to silicone, but no clinical roles or biological effects on resistance to infection, tumor surveillance or immune responses have been demonstrated in these studies.

Evidence for a particular HLA (human lymphocyte antigen) class I or class II haplotype associated with symptomatic women with silicone breast implants, or for specific T-cell activation or delayed hypersensitivity to silicone is insufficient and often flawed, and there is limited evidence that HLA haplotypes of symptomatic women with implants resemble those of symptomatic women without implants and that there is no T-cell activation or delayed hypersensitivity from silicone. Studies addressing these issues are limited and technical problems substantial, providing the committee with no support for a role of silicone as a T-cell antigen or in creating T-cell autoantigens. The committee also finds no evidence for antisilicone antibodies. The clinical significance of a recently described antipolymer antibody test is unclear, although the polymer in question is not silicone or silicon containing, and it is extremely unlikely that it measures an antisilicone antibody. The committee also noted several reports suggesting that women with breast implants might have elevated serum immunoglobulin levels. A few case reports also suggested that there might be an increased frequency of multiple myeloma in women with breast implants. These data are insufficient and a number of current epidemiological studies do not report an increase in immunoglobulin levels or multiple myeloma in such women.

Reports of antinuclear antibodies and epidemiological studies of classical and atypical connective tissue or rheumatic disease in women with breast implants also do not provide any support for immunologic or autoimmune responses or diseases associated with silicone breast implants.

The committee reviewed 30 studies of antinuclear antibodies and other autoantibodies in women with silicone (primarily gel-filled) breast implants.

These reports were often conflicting; many used differing technologies to assay antinuclear antibodies or differing criteria to determine a positive test. Lack of controls and other design problems hampered the interpretation of some studies. No pattern of association of antinuclear antibodies with silicone breast implants emerged from these data. Several epidemiological studies suggested support for the conclusion that there is no association of antinuclear or other autoantibodies with breast implants.

A review of 17 epidemiological reports of connective tissue disease in women with breast implants was remarkable for the consistency in finding no elevated relative risk or odds ratio for an association of implants with disease. Studies of breast implants and undifferentiated connective tissue disease or atypical signs and symptoms were much fewer in number. Several high-quality studies of classical connective tissue disease in women with implants were available, but this was not the case with atypical signs and symptoms or unusual presentations. Nevertheless, many of the studies focusing on classical disease had also collected data on rheumatic and related signs and symptoms, and in general, no association with implants was found. A novel syndrome or disease associated with silicone breast implants has been proposed. Evidence for this proposed disease rests on case reports and is insufficient or flawed. The disease definition includes, as a precondition, the presence of silicone breast implants, so it cannot be studied as an independent health problem. The committee finds that the diagnosis of this condition could depend on the presence of a number of symptoms that are nonspecific and common in the general population.

Thus, there does not appear to be even suggestive evidence for the existence of a novel syndrome in women with breast implants. In fact, epidemiological evidence suggests that there is no novel syndrome.

Silicone like many polymers (and other substances) can cause solid state carcinogenesis. Implantation of a material formulated with appropriate size, shape, and surface characteristics causes infrequently metastasizing sarcomas in susceptible rodent species. This phenomenon is not believed to occur in humans, and no increases in human breast sarcomas have been observed. Epidemiological studies have not found elevated relative risks for breast cancer in women with implants. In fact, some of these studies, now evaluating women two decades or more after implantation, have found fewer breast cancers than expected, and some animal studies have suggested that breast implants might be associated with lower frequencies of breast cancer. The committee cannot find that evidence for a lower risk of breast cancer in women with breast implants is conclusive, but the committee does conclude that there is no increase in primary or recurrent breast cancer in these women.

Occasional reports of cancer occurring in the breasts of women injected with silicone for breast augmentation have been noted . . . but these are uncontrolled case reports or anecdotes, and do not constitute useful evidence of any carcinogenic effect of silicone in humans. Several cohort studies have examined the risk for all cancers combined in women with breast implants, and all have reported numbers of cases similar to or lower than the number expected based on rates in the general population. The committee concludes that evidence is lacking for a relationship of breast implants to any specific cancers. Neurologic disease, symptoms, and pathological and physical findings have been reported in case series of women with breast implants by a few groups. Other investigators have not found neurological problems and have criticized the experimental design used in reports of such an association. Experimental animal studies do not lend support to silicone as a cause of neurologic disease. Some case reports describe silicone gel deposits that migrate from ruptured breast implants, causing scarring and constriction around peripheral nerves. However, reports that silicone might be associated with autoantibodies to nerve components, that silica might be present in the nerves of women with implants, or that multiple sclerosis-like or other neurologic syndromes might be associated with implants have been found to have design and methodological problems that limited any conclusions. Two epidemiological studies of neurologic disease in women with implants provide limited support for a conclusion that there is no elevated relative risk for any association, and the committee concludes that with the exception of local problems caused by the migration of gel from ruptured implants, evidence that silicone breast implants cause neurologic signs, symptoms, or disease is lacking or flawed.

In an overall consideration of the epidemiological evidence, the committee noted that because there are more than 1.5 million adult women of all ages in the United States with silicone breast implants, some of these women would be expected to develop connective tissue diseases, cancer, neurological diseases, or other systemic complaints or conditions. Evidence suggests that such diseases or conditions are no more common in women with breast implants than in women without implants.

A few investigators have proposed that women with silicone breast implants might transmit silicone or some immunological factor via breast milk or across the placenta to their children. There is limited evidence that implantation, especially through a periareolar incision, may interfere with lactation and breast feeding, but no differences are observed in milk or blood silicon (and thus presumably silicone) levels in lactating women with implants compared to lactating control women without implants.

Much higher levels of silicon have been measured in cows' milk at the retail level and commercially available infant formula. It is likely that some of this silicon is organic. Infants are also exposed to other sources of silicone, for example, pacifiers, nipples, and widely available drops for colic. Antinuclear antibodies are reported in normal women without implants, and no untoward effects on their children have been observed.

The committee can find no evidence of elevated silicone in breast milk or of any other substance that would be deleterious to infants. Because there is conclusive evidence that breast feeding is beneficial to infants, the committee strongly recommends a trial of breast feeding by mothers with implants.

A single group of investigators examined children at about 5 years of age who had been breast fed by mothers with implants and reported abnormalities of esophageal motility that they hypothesized might have been caused by exposure to silicone. . . . .

The committee concludes that evidence for health effects in children related to maternal breast implants is insufficient or flawed. Breast implants interfere with diagnostic and screening imaging examinations of the breast by compressing and distorting breast tissue, by making compression of the breast in a mammographic examination difficult and obligating special views, and by interposing (particularly with gel-filled implants) a radiopaque mass in the middle of the breast that obscures some breast tissue. These problems are fewer with submuscular placement of the implant and can be at least partially overcome with special views. Data on whether cancer detection is impaired by implants do not allow definite conclusions, but no studies have shown increases in cancer mortality in women with implants because of diagnostic delays. Mammographic screening for cancer in women with implants under the same conditions as recommended for women without implants should be encouraged.

. . . . Magnetic resonance imaging is the most sensitive and specific technology for rupture diagnosis. The committee did not find direct evidence on the cost/benefit of screening for rupture, however. Relevant screening data and analysis might allow a firmer conclusion on screening in general or in women with implants with known high prevalence of rupture or in other specific circumstances. Only if such data showed reduced morbidity as a result of screening and a screening driven intervention, would routine screening of the general population of asymptomatic women with breast implants be justified.

Conclusions and Research Recommendations

The committee wishes to highlight the following conclusions from this Summary:

- There is extensive presence of, and wide exposure of citizens of developed countries to silicones in foods, cosmetics, lubricants for machinery, hypodermic syringes and other products, insulators and a wide array of consumer products.
- The committee concludes that a review of the toxicology studies of silicones and other substances known to be in breast implants does not provide a basis for health concerns.

The committee has reached three major conclusions regarding local and perioperative complications. First, reoperations and local and perioperative complications are frequent enough to be a cause for concern and to justify the conclusion that they are the primary safety issue with silicone breast implants. Complications may have risks themselves, such as pain, disfigurement and serious infection and they may lead to medical and surgical interventions, such as reoperations, that have risks. Second, risks accumulate over the lifetime of the implant, but quantitative data on this point are lacking for modern implants and deficient historically.

Third, information concerning the nature and the relatively high frequency of local complications and reoperations is an essential element of adequate informed consent for women undergoing breast implantation.

The committee has also come to the following conclusions:

- Studies addressing the immunology of silicones are limited and technical problems substantial, providing the committee with no support for an immunologic role of silicone.
- A novel syndrome or disease associated with silicone breast implants has been proposed by a small group of physicians. Evidence for this proposed disease rests on case reports and is insufficient and flawed. The disease definition includes, as a precondition, the presence of silicone gel breast implants, so it cannot be studied as an independent health problem. The committee finds that the diagnosis of this condition could depend on the presence of a number of symptoms that are nonspecific and common in the general population. Thus, there does not appear to be even suggestive evidence of a novel syndrome in women with breast implants. In fact, epidemiological evidence suggests that there is no novel syndrome.
- There is no increase in primary or recurrent breast cancer in implanted women.
- In an overall consideration of the epidemiological evidence, the committee noted that because there are more than 1.5 million adult women of all ages in the United States with silicone breast implants, some of these women would be expected to develop connective tissue diseases, cancer, neurological diseases or other systemic complaints or conditions. Evidence suggests that such diseases or conditions are no more common in women with breast implants than in women without implants.
- The committee finds no evidence of elevated silicone in breast milk or any other substance that would be deleterious to infants; the committee strongly concludes that all mothers with implants should attempt breast feeding.

- The committee concludes that evidence for health effects in children related to maternal breast implants is insufficient or flawed.

Recommendations for Research

1. Reliable techniques for the measuring of silicone concentrations in body fluids and tissues are needed to provide established, agreed-upon values and ranges of silicone concentrations in body fluids and tissues with or without exposure to silicone from an implanted medical device. Such developments could improve the study of silicones and silicone distribution in humans, could help with regulatory requirements, and might in some circumstances resolve questions by providing quantitative data on the presence or absence of silicones.
2. Ongoing surveillance of recipients of silicone breast implants should be carried out for representative groups of women, including long term outcomes and local complications, with attention to, or definition of the following:
   - implant physical and chemical characteristics,
   - tracking identified individual implants,
   - using appropriate, standardized, and validated technologies for detecting and defining outcomes,
   - carrying out associated toxicology studies by standards consistent with accepted toxicological standards for other devices; and
   - ensuring representative samples, appropriate controls and randomization in any specific studies, as required by good experimental design.
3. The development of a national model of informed consent for women undergoing breast implantation should be encouraged, and the

3: FDA Press Release, 2006

The following statement from the FDA assured some people that implants are safe.

Source: "FDA Approves Silicone Gel-Filled Breast Implants after In-Depth Evaluation Agency Requiring 10 Years of Patient Follow-Up." FDA News Release, 2006. Available: http://www.natap.org/2006/newsUpdates/120406_11.htm. Accessed July 27, 2011.

FDA News Release

FOR IMMEDIATE RELEASE P06–189
November 17, 2006 **Media Inquiries:** Heidi Valetkevitch, 301–827–6242
Consumer Inquiries: 888-INFO-FDA

FDA Approves Silicone Gel-Filled Breast Implants after In-Depth Evaluation Agency Requiring 10 Years of Patient Follow-Up

After rigorous scientific review, the U.S. Food and Drug Administration (FDA) today approved the marketing of silicone gel-filled breast implants made by two companies for breast reconstruction in women of all ages and breast augmentation in women ages 22 and older. The products are manufactured by Allergan Corp. (formerly Inamed Corp.), Irvine, Calif., and Mentor Corp., Santa Barbara, Calif.

"FDA has reviewed an extensive amount of data from clinical trials of women studied for up to four years, as well as a wealth of other information to determine the benefits and risks of these products," said Daniel Schultz, M.D., Director, Center for Devices and Radiological Health, FDA. "The extensive body of scientific evidence provides reasonable assurance of the benefits and risks of these devices. This information is available in the product labeling and will enable women and their physicians to make informed decisions."

Now that the products have been determined to be safe and effective, FDA will continue to monitor them by requiring each company to conduct a large postapproval study following about 40,000 women for 10 years after receiving breast implants. FDA often requires postmarket studies to answer important questions that can only be answered once a product is in broader use, such as the incidence of rare adverse events.

FDA's decision to approve these implants was based on a thorough review of each company's clinical (core) and preclinical studies, a review of studies by independent scientific bodies and deliberations of advisory panels of outside experts that heard public comment from hundreds of stakeholders. In addition, FDA conducted inspections of each company's manufacturing facilities to determine that they comply with FDA's Good Manufacturing Practices. Some of the complications reported in the core studies included hardening of the area around the implant, breast pain, change in nipple sensation, implant rupture and the need for additional surgery. However, the majority of women in these studies reported being satisfied with their implants.

In the past decade, a number of independent studies have examined whether silicone gel-filled breast implants are associated with connective tissue disease or cancer. The studies, including a report by the Institute of Medicine, have concluded there is no convincing evidence that breast implants are associated with either of these diseases. However, these issues will be addressed further in the postapproval studies conducted by the companies.

"The silicone breast implant is one of the most extensively studied medical devices," said Schultz. "We now have a good understanding of what complications can occur and at what rates. We also know that women who get these devices will probably need to have additional breast implant surgery at least once. This is valuable information for women who may be considering these products."

Full information about the risks and benefits of the devices can be found in the package and patient labeling mandated by FDA. The patient labeling outlines some of the important factors women should consider when deciding whether to get silicone gel-filled breast implants. Some of these factors are: breast implants are not lifetime devices and a woman will likely need additional surgeries on her breast at least once over her lifetime; many of the changes to a woman's breast following implantation are irreversible; rupture of a silicone gel-filled breast implant is most often silent, which means that usually neither the woman nor her surgeon will know that her implants have ruptured; and a woman will need regular screening MRI examinations over her lifetime to determine if silent rupture has occurred. The device labeling states that a woman should have her first MRI three years after her initial implant surgery and then every two years thereafter. The cost of MRI screening over a woman's lifetime may exceed the cost of her initial surgery and may not be covered by medical insurance. The labeling also states that if implant rupture is noted on an MRI, the implant should be removed and replaced, if needed.

FDA approved the silicone gel-filled breast implants with a number of conditions, including requiring each company to: conduct a large postapproval study; continue its core study through 10 years; conduct a focus group study of the patient labeling; continue laboratory studies to further characterize types of device failure; and track each implant in the event, for example, that health professionals and patients need to be notified of updated product information.

The postapproval studies will continue to gather information about the safety and effectiveness of the implants. Information will be collected about rates of local complications, rates of connective tissue disease and its signs and symptoms, rates of neurological disease and its signs and symptoms, potential effects on offspring of women with breast implants, potential effects on reproduction and lactation, rates of cancer, rates of suicide, potential interference of breast implants with mammography, and MRI compliance and rupture rates.

The postapproval studies will be closely monitored by FDA. FDA anticipates that data from the studies will provide important information for patients and physicians, and may lead to improvements in device labeling.

For more information, visit www.fda.gov/cdrh/breastimplants

4: Position Statement on Cosmetic Surgery for Children with Down Syndrome, 2011

When families are faced with the options about medical care for their children with Down syndrome, they often find so many opinions that they are conflicted or confused regarding what, if anything, they should do about the appearance of their child. The following position statement from the National Down Syndrome Society provides some guidance.

The decision to have cosmetic surgery is always a personal one, and the National Down Syndrome Society supports people with Down syndrome and their families in their individual choices. However, the National Down Syndrome Society (NDSS) believes that such a decision should be an informed one, made by the family with the help of doctors, counselors, and other interested parties.

For 20 years, NDSS has worked for inclusion and acceptance for all people with Down syndrome. Today more than ever, people with Down syndrome learn in regular classrooms, are employed in a variety of jobs, and interact in many different ways in the larger community. NDSS believes in supporting individuals with Down syndrome through full inclusion in the community and by not attaching a stigma to their physical features.

The goal of inclusion and acceptance is mutual respect based on who we are as individuals, not how we look. Altering a child's appearance as a means of encouraging acceptance does not change the reality of the disability. In fact, some education experts believe that the physical characteristics of Down syndrome may offer visual cues to people about an individual's disability and thus foster an easier acceptance and understanding of that disability. Many families believe that to alter their child's facial features would be to disrespect his or her individuality and that an important part of that individuality is the condition of Down syndrome.

It should be noted that cosmetic surgery is performed on a very small number of people with Down syndrome. NDSS advises parents considering cosmetic surgery to become educated about all aspects of the procedure as well as the physical, social and psychological consequences for their child, and to make an informed decision based on this knowledge.

Plastic Surgery Time Line

The following is a chronology of significant events in the history of plastic surgery.

800 BCE   Skin grafts are used in India. The Edwin Smith Papyrus states that the technique of suturing was used. This surgical papyrus, written in the 17th century BCE, is based on healing principles from 3000 BCE. Edwin Smith, an Egyptologist, discovered it in Luxor and purchased it from unscrupulous individuals. He was unable to translate it completely. After he died, his daughter donated the 17-page document to the New York Historical Society where it was later translated in full by Henry Breasted in 1930. The writings consist of case histories of 48 individuals.

Rhinoplasties are performed in India for adulterers.

131–201 CE   Galen (129–199) writes *De Faciis,* a treatise about craniofacial surgery and how to apply bandages to the wounds.

1140   King Ruggiero, in Salerno, Italy, issues an edit that requires aspiring surgeons to undergo examinations at the Scuola Salernitana.

1308   Richard the Barber forms a group to discourage conduct that "could bring discredit upon the profession"(Santoni-Rugui and Sykes 2007, 58).

1346   Military surgeon recruited to treat the wounded in the battle of Ypres.

1349   In Italy, Florence physicians form a guild for its members with strict standards for taking courses and attending dissections.

1497   First treatise on surgery, *Dis est das Buch der Chirurgia Hautwirkung der Wundartsney*, written by Hieronymous Brunschwig (1450–1512).

1572 Ambröise Paré (1510–1590) publishes the first scientific text in Paris, France, a book about battlefield injuries and burns.

Renaissance Germany: Wilhelm Fabrey von Hilden (1650–1624) writes a book on burns called *Traumi Termici*. He divides burns into three categories: levissim (redness and moderate pain); mediocrem (marked pain, swelling and blisters); and insignam (skin necrosis). He introduces healing aids such as splints to minimize contraction and pieces of cloth to keep eyelid or lip skin from forming adhesions with adjoining tissues.

Italy: Noses are rebuilt on syphilitic patients. Gaspare Tagliacozzi (1545–1599) rediscovers ancient technique of skin flaps used by Susruta in India, the Brancas in Sicily, and the Vianeos in Calabria. He experiments with skin grafts using skin tissue from the forearm for the donor site.

1660 U.K. Royal Society founded in London.

1730 France: Academie Nationale de Medicine founded.

1798 France: Pierre Joseph Desault, a French anatomist, coins the term "plastic surgery."

1799 France: Francois Chopart (1743–1795) employs a pedicle flap to close a lip injury.

1818 Germany: Karl Ferdinand von Gräefe publishes *Rhinoplastic,* a monograph on plastic surgery of the nose. and revises Tagliacozzi's method by using skin from the forehead instead of the upper arm. Immediately afterward, a flurry of new "plasties" on other parts of the body are tried.

1826 Johann Friedrich Dieffenbach (Germany) is the first surgeon to successfully close a cleft palate.

1827 Virginia, United States: John Peter Mettauer (1787–1875) performs the first cleft palate operation in the New World with self-designed instruments.

1895 *Clostridium botulinum* is isolated from food and postmortem tissues by Emile Van Ermengem.

1915 Dr. Varaztad H. Kazanjian (1879–1974) establishes the first dental and maxillofacial unit clinic in France as part of Harvard University's services at the General Hospital in Camiers. The clinic eventually moves to enlarged facilities and continues until 1919. Dr. Kazanjian treats approximately 3,000 patients and is dubbed "Miracle Man of the Western Front."

1921 Three surgeons meet in Chicago and elect 20 surgeons as founding members of the American Association of Oral Surgeons.

Membership requires both dental and medical degrees; however, two exceptions are made: Chalmers Lyons, who had a dental degree only, and Vilray Blair, who had a medical degree only.

1923 The requirement for a dual degree is dropped. Those with medical degrees no longer had to acquire a dental degree.

1925 Jacques Maliniac and Gustave Aufricht open a private practice and persuade the City Hospital in New York to open a plastic surgery division.

1931 Jacques Maliniac establishes the Society of Plastic and Reconstructive Surgery with colleagues Clarence Straatsma and Lyon Peer as charter members. Four are board certified otolaryngologists and one is an ophthalmologist.

1937 The American Association of Oral Surgeons' name is broadened to the American Association of Oral and Plastic Surgeons.

1937 The American Association of Oral and Plastic Surgeons enlarges its mission to include formal training programs. It creates the American Board of Plastic Surgery to establish standards for certification in plastic surgery.

1939 The Dermatome is invented. It calibrates split thickness skin grafts.

early 1940s The Society of Plastic and Reconstructive Surgery changes its name to the American Society of Plastic and Reconstructive Surgeons (ASPRS).

1941 The American Medical Association's Advisory Board of Medical Specialties admits the American Board of Plastic Surgery as a new specialty.

1942 The American Association of Oral and Plastic Surgeons changes its name to the American Association of Plastic Surgeons.

1946 Gustav Aufricht and the publisher Williams and Wilkins launch the *Journal of Plastic and Reconstructive Surgery,* the official journal for the American Society of Plastic Surgeons (ASPS). Edward Schantz purifies the *Clostridium botulinum* toxin in crystalline form for potential biological warfare.

1949 *The Surgical Treatment of Facial Injuries* by Kazanjians and John M. Converse is published. It is considered a classic work in the field of plastic surgery.

1949 Member surgeons number 150. Jacques Maliniac forms the Educational Foundation of the ASPS now known as the Plastic Surgery Educational Foundation (PSEF). Its mission is to send American surgeons to Third World nations to help train physicians who would otherwise not have access to advanced surgical techniques.

1950s   Plastic surgery is now integrated into the American health care system. As a result of emergency situations during wartime, internal wiring for facial fractures, rotation flaps for skin deformities, and other innovations are developed.

1954   Dr. Joseph Murray performs the world's first successful kidney transplant.

1959   Murray performs the world's first successful allograft.

1960s   Silicone emerges as a new tool to use in breast implants.

1962   Murray performs the first cadaveric renal transplant.

1969   Hal B. Jennings, a plastic surgeon, is appointed Surgeon General of the United States.

1970s   Alan Scott investigates nonsurgical methods for squinting with *C. botulinum*.

1970   George Crikelair, concerned because of the number of pediatric burns, develops flame-retardant children's sleepwear and clothing.

1972   The National Archives of Plastic Surgery is established by Boston plastic surgeon Dr. Robert Goldwyn, and placed in the Francis A. Countway Library of Medicine. The archives is sponsored by The American Society of Plastic Surgeons, The Plastic Surgery Educational Foundation, The American Association of Plastic Surgeons, The American Society for Aesthetic Plastic Surgery, and The American Society of Maxillofacial Surgeons. The Archives' goal is to acquire, preserve, and make available material that records the development of plastic and reconstructive surgery by collecting the official records, correspondence, minutes of meetings, photographs, and films of professional organizations and the personal papers of distinguished plastic surgeons.

1980s   ASPS produces informational brochures for the public. Members display these brochures in their offices for patients to read regarding their potential surgery.

1987   Jean Carruthers observes that Botox used to treat blepharospasm obliterates frown lines.

1989   FDA approves Botox for strabismus and facial spasms.

1992   Carruthers publishes a paper that describes Botox application for ablation of frown lines.

1996   ASPRS launches the Plastic Surgery Education Campaign, an awareness campaign that seeks to educate the public on the importance of choosing a board-certified plastic surgeon.

1998   President Clinton signs a bill to require insurance companies to cover the cost of reconstructive breast surgery for women who have undergone a mastectomy.

1999 The American Society of Plastic and Reconstructive Surgeons changes its name to the American Society of Plastic Surgeons (ASPS).

1999 Florida's State Board of Medicine declares a 90-day moratorium on office-based liposuction combined with abdominoplasty after newspapers publish articles about 10 patients who died after undergoing cosmetic procedures.

ASPS forms the Task Force on Patient Safety and Office-Based Surgery Facilities to review and evaluate risk factors.

2000 The ASPS board of directors amends its bylaws to require all members performing surgery under anesthesia to do so in only accredited, licensed, or Medicare-certified surgical facilities.

2000 After the ABC television network asks ASPS to allow its members to participate in the show *Extreme Makeover,* the society's executive committee consents with the stipulation that the doctor-patient relationship is not lost and the patient selection does not devolve into a contest.

2002 All members of the ASPS who perform surgery under anesthesia can do so only in accredited, licensed, or Medicare-certified surgical facilities.

2002 The FDA approves Botox for medical procedures such as wrinkle removal and frown-line injections.

2003 More than 8.7 million cosmetic procedures are performed.

2004 14.8 million plastic surgery procedures are performed in the United States.

2005 The FDA grants silicone implants the status of "approvable with conditions."

2006 16.2 million plastic surgery procedures are performed in the United States.

2006 The FDA approves silicone implants for general patient use.

REFERENCES AND FURTHER READING

Fox, Claire, and William P. Graham. 1988. *The American Board of Plastic Surgery, 1937–1987.* Reprinted from *Plastic and Reconstructive Surgery.*

Santoni-Rugui, Paolo and Phillip Sykes. 2007. *A History of Plastic Surgery.* Heidelberg: Springer-Verlag.

Glossary

The following terms are included to define words used in Internet advertising and in this book. Patients need to know what the words in a brochure mean, especially if one is considering undergoing any kind of medical or surgical procedure.

Abdominoplasty—commonly called a "tummy tuck." It involves cutting the abdominal skin from hip to hip, creating a flap. The flap is raised and the excess abdominal skin is removed. Sometimes, liposuction is performed during the surgery. Abdominoplasty is one of the most common plastic surgery procedures chosen by patients. There are a number of different incisions that are made. The "French cut" is made lower in the pelvis so that a bikini bathing suit will not reveal the scar. According to the American Board of Plastic Surgery, in 2009,115,191 people had an abdominoplasty. There are at least 15 types of incision styles used to remove abdominal fat on obese individuals or pendulous abdomens.[1]

Acculift instant facelift—a new nonsurgical facelift, as advertised by a number of plastic surgeons on the Internet. It uses laser-assisted lipolysis (fat destruction) and will take away excess fat from the face but not remove wrinkles. It is not a substitute for a facelift or a mini-lift but it is a minimal procedure that will provide satisfactory results.

AcHyal—one brand name for hyaluronic acid used as a filler or treatment for acne. Other brands are Hylaform, Restylane, Perlane, Juvederm, Rofilan Hylan, and Hylaform plus.

Allograft—a graft transplanted between genetically nonidentical individuals of the same species.

Alpha hydroxy acid (AHA)—one substance used for a chemical peel. The mildest peels are those that use AHA, which include glycolic, lactic, or citric acid. No anesthesia is needed. The patient feels a mild stinging or tingling sensation. AHA can be mixed with other substances to use as a home treatment. With this mildest of the peels, the patient may need additional treatments.

Ambiguous—difficult to determine; in this book, refers to sexual organs of a newborn baby that do not conform to the expected size and shape of a biological male or a biological female.

Anomaly—a physical characteristic that is not usual or normal, such as a sixth finger or fused toes.

Areola—the pigmented portion of the breast surrounding the nipple.

Augmentation Mammaplasty—(also spelled mammoplasty) the operation that women undergo to enlarge the size of their breasts. It consists of inserting saline-filled implants, either under the skin or under the pectoral muscle. Previous implants were made with silicone gel but controversy regarding their safety led to the development of using sterile saline, instead. The operation is performed under general anesthesia. There have been deaths resulting from this procedure performed with local anesthesia because so much was required to deaden the operating field.

Autograft—tissue or organ transferred to a new position in the body of the same individual

Autologous fat injection—fat from the patient can be used to fill in defects and smooth out large contours but not fine wrinkles. Unfortunately, the fat resorbs within 6 to 12 months after the procedure. Commonly used donor sites are the abdomen, buttocks, thighs, and under the chin.

Blepharoplasty—surgery that removes fatty tissue and loose skin from the upper and lower eyelids.

Board Certified—a requirement for a physician to have completed a certain number of procedures in order to have this title.

Body contouring—a combination of procedures such as liposuction, lifts, fills, and implants to shape the body to a desired form.

Body lift—surgical procedures to correct abdomen, buttocks, or other places of the body that have sagged as a result of aging.

Botox–brand name for Botulinum toxin which is used to paralyze the facial muscles that cause frown lines.

Bovine collagen—collagen made from cows. A few brand names of bovine collagen are Restoplast®, Zyplast®, and Zyderm®.

Bridalplasty—a reality TV program that stresses beauty as the epitome of values.

Brow lift—reduces creases and frown lines. Correct droopy eyebrows that create hoods over the eyes. This is often performed as part of a facelift.

Chemical peels—the application of a chemical to the facial skin, which has been sun damaged, wrinkled, or is unevenly pigmented. AHA, TCA, and Phenol are used for various degrees of chemical skin peels, AHA being the mildest and Phenol the strongest. These are nonsurgical procedures that require variable amounts of time, depending on which chemical is used and how extensive its application.

Cleft palate—technically known as palatoschisis, a condition often associated with a hare lip that results from an incomplete closure of the palate. Surgery is necessary so that the newborn does not aspirate milk. A second surgery will be required prior to the acquisition of language so that the child does not have a nasal sound to his or her speech.

Collagen injections—Collagen is a protein found in animal tissues. When aging results in weakened connective tissue that sags and forms lines, injections are used to smooth out lip lines, smile lines, frown lines, and other unwanted facial lines. Collagen from cows is called bovine collagen and was approved for plastic surgery use in 1981. It is not recommended for use near the eyes or into the lips. Problems may result if a local anesthetic is used instead of a topical anesthetic because the liquid anesthetic becomes incorporated with the collagen being injected and distorts the injection site. Human collagen brands include Dermalogen®, Cymetra®, CosmoPlast®, and CosmoDerm®.

Columella—the horizontal cartilage between the nostrils and above the philtrum.

Composite graft—a graft composed of several layers of tissue such as skin and cartilage.

Congenital—born with a certain disability or anomaly that is either genetic (inborn) or the result of physical, chemical, or environmental damage that occurred while in utero.

Contracture—muscle shortening because of spasm or loss of muscular balance.

Cosmetic surgery—surgery to enhance a person's appearance, elective.

Cosmetic surgery tourism—an incentive offered by European, Asian, and South American countries where a patient buys airfare, hotel, hospital, doctor, and anesthesia to have a procedure at much less the cost than they would pay in the United States.

Crescent mastopexy—the minimal mastopexy technique and involves removing a small crescent-shaped piece of skin above the areola, which leaves a small scar above the nipple.

Cryosurgery—spraying and freezing the skin with liquid nitrogen, used for removing small skin growths.

Curettage—a process where an instrument is used to scrape tissue. A curette looks like a small spoon with its center removed so that the inside edges are razor sharp. The handle is long and allows the operator to work at a distance so that the operating field is not obscured by his or her hands.

Cutaneous—related to the skin.

Dermabrasion—a way to remove or improve scars on the face. It is also referred to as surgical skin planing. The patient is given a local anesthetic injection to numb the skin and then uses a tool to "sand the skin."

Donut mastopexy (Benelli mastopexy)—this breast lift is performed on more extensive breast falling than the crescent technique is used for. The donut mastopexy moves the nipple higher by cutting around the areola and removing a donut-shaped piece of skin. The scar resembles a donut because it is circumareolar.

Edema—swelling caused by the accumulation of fluid in tissues.

Embolism—an impediment to the flow of blood, by a blood clot or fat.

Emulsify—to break up in small pieces as is done in ultrasonicliposuction.

Epicanthic—the eyefold above the eye and in the inner corner of the eye. Asian people have a prominent epicanthic eyefold and sometimes request that it be removed so that their eye looks rounder (and less Asian).

Epinephrine—an extract from the medulla of the adrenal glands. It has two uses in medicine: one as a stimulant, to revive a stopped heart and the other to stop bleeding. It is used in tumescent liposuction, along with the Lidocaine to constrict the blood vessels so that the patient does not bleed.

Escharotomy—surgery to correct the constriction caused by a scar.

Extreme Makeover—a former reality ABC TV program, similar to *The Swan*.

Facelifts—a group of procedures which, combined, remove signs of aging such as sagging skin, double chin, wrinkles, frown lines, and excessive fat pads. Sometimes, cheek or chin implants are inserted.

Flap—skin that is first dissected from the underlying layers and then moved to cover another adjacent part of the body.

Forehead lift—usually performed in conjunction with brow lift.

Free flap—flap in which the donor blood vessels are severed and the tissue is moved to another part of the body, then reconnected with the vessels in that part.

Gender—the masculine or feminine gestures, way of dressing, acting, and relating. It is a construct rather than a biological fact. Gender and sex are often used interchangeably but they do not mean the same thing.

Genitalia—the external sexual organs.

Gonad—internal sex organs such as ovaries and testicles before they descend.

Graft—skin that is transplanted from one part of the body to another to repair a defect.

Hyalouronic acid—this is a non-surgical treatment, a temporary filler used to soften facial lines and furrows. It is used to soften glabellar lines (frown lines), perioral lines (smokers lines, vertical lines on the mouth), oral commisures (Marionette lines that form at the corner of the mouth), forehead lines, periorbital lines (lines around the eyes, Crow's feet), nasolabial furrows (deep smile lines), cheek depressions, acne scars, and minor facial scars. It is used instead of collagen because it is non-allergenic. Collagen is made from bovine (cow) protein and some people are allergic to it.

Hyperpigmentation—redness or extra color to the skin that does not match the rest.

Hypertrophy—overgrowth. An hypertrophic scar is called a keloid and often forms on individuals of African American heritage.

I Want a Famous Face—A former reality MTV program where individuals had plastic surgery elsewhere and then presented themselves to the TV audience with their narratives about why they wanted to look like a particular celebrity or other person.

Incision—a cut that is made in the place where surgery first begins.

Injectable subsurface augmentation—materials like collagen and the patient's own fat which are injected into areas that need to be smoothed out or filled in. The autmentation is not always permanent and may need to be repeated.

Laser—an acronym for light amplification by stimulated emission of radiation. A laser is used for certain types of surgery instead of a scalpel. In plastic surgery, a laser is used to cut, seal, or vaporize skin and blood vessels. Laser therapy is used to rejuvenate aging and sun-damaged skin. Laser therapy also eliminates spider veins. Laser resurfacing is used to change the surface of the skin so that new skin will grow at the scar site.

Lateral—toward the side.

Lidocaine—a local anesthetic that is used for plastic surgery in small areas. It is similar to the novocaine that dentists use. In tumescent liposuction, Lidocaine is mixed with saline and injected into the area before removing the fat.

Lip augmentation—collagen or hyaluronic acid injections are used to make the lips plumper. It is not a permanent change. The procedure will need to be redone every few months.

Lipoma—a benign fatty tumor.

Lipoplasty—liposuction.

Liposuction—A procedure that uses a cannula and suction to remove fat from the body. Also called suction lipectomy.

Lite-laser—a laser technique also referred to as "cold laser."

Lollipop breast lift—a type of mastopexy for the most severe or pronounced breast droopiness. The skin is removed around the areola and the lower part of the breast. The surgery is referred to as "lollipop," because the scar resembles a lollipop.

Lower body lift—also known as a belt lipectomy. The surgery is usually performed after massive weight loss when there is redundant skin and tissue in the lower abdomen, hips, and flank. Fat and skin are removed first, then the shape of the lower body is recontoured.

Malar augmentation—cheek implant.

Mandible—the lower jaw.

Mastopexy—this is also called a breast lift. It is done for women who do not want implants but want to raise sagging breasts. There are three types of mastopexy: crescent, donut, and lollipop. The above the nipple and the skin is pulled until the height of the In 2009, 87,396 mastopexies were performed in the United States.

Maxilla—the upper jaw.

Medial—toward the middle.

Melanoma—the most serious skin cancer, also called malignant melanoma that spreads to other body tissues because it occurs in the deepest portion of the skin.

Microdermabrasion—noninvasive skin care process that exfoliates and resurfaces the skin, one layer at a time. The chemicals used are aluminum or salt crystals. Sun damage, fine lines and wrinkles, rough skin, age spots, and irregular pigmentation respond to this type of treatment.

Moh's chemosurgery or Moh's microsurgery—this surgery is performed in stages. As each thin piece of tissue is removed, it is frozen so that the lab can look at the histology. After anesthetic is injected, the doctor curettes the tumor to assess its horizontal and vertical extent. The surgery begins with a 45-degree angle incision, which goes around the clinical margins of the specimen. The specimen is removed and divided into four equal quadrants. Then each quadrant is marked with two different color dyes. The doctor will mark the tissue sample to indicate its orientation (skin edge versus subcutaneous layer). In the lab, the technician will cut and stain the sections. Moh's differs from other surgery because the samples it takes are horizontal rather than "bread-loaf" and include the side and deep margins. When the sample of each part no longer shows residual pathology, the surgery stops. A flap or graft is sometimes needed after surgery. The advantage of Moh's over other surgical methods is that Moh's is tissue sparing. As soon as the margins are free from disease, the surgery is over. Moh's can be used cosmetically and functionally in important areas. In addition to the face and nose, Moh's is used for genital, anal, perianal, hand, foot and nail areas. It is indicated when there is a recurrent or incompletely removed basal cell or squamous cell carcinoma, in rapidly growing tumors that are greater than 2 centimeters (approximately 1 inch).

Nasolabial fold—the crease that appears as a result of aging between the nose and the mouth.

Necrosis—tissue death and decay. Necrotic tissue is usually blackish and horribly odoriferous.

Nevus, nevi—mole or moles, pigmented growths on the skin that can be removed with ethyl chloride or cauterization.

Nonablative laser treatment—uses an intense beam of light to stimulate the production of collagen without going through the outer layer of skin.

Nonsurgical facial rejuvenation—any of a number of procedures either alone or in combination that improves the appearance of the face without surgical intervention.

Obturator—a device used to help a child with a cleft lip eat or drink prior to surgery to repair the defect. The obturator is warn inside the mouth and maintains the arch necessary for ease in eating.

Otoplasty—a surgical procedure to reposition or reshape the ear. Often performed on children whose ears stick out.

Pectoral implants—implants used to make the chest muscle appear more developed, usually for men.

Perineum—the area of the body between the rectum and the labia in a female, and between the rectum and the scrotum in a male.

Philtrum—the space between the bottom of the nose and the top of the lip.

Plasty—the suffix that indicates a plastic surgery operation.

PMMA—a synthetic implant material that consists of tiny particles suspended in collagen gel to get rid of wrinkles. One brand name of PMMA is Artecoll®.

Redundant—extra.

Reparative surgery—surgery necessary to fix or restore function.

Reduction mammaplasty—a surgical procedure to reduce the size of the breasts.

Restylane—this is a chemical called hyaluronic acid used to plump up areas of the face which lips, nasal folds or other depressions caused by scars. It is advertised to smoothing wrinkles and folds around the mouth. The way it works is by binding with water. The results are instant but only last for a few months. There may be swelling and tenderness in the areas of the injections. It is approved by the FDA.

Rhytidectomy—a facelift that includes various techniques such as brow lift, jowl removal, cheek implants, forehead lift, wrinkle removal, blepharoplasty and collagen, PMMA, or hyaluronic acid fillers.

Saline implants—breast implants that replaced the former popular silicone implants because of controversial issues regarding silicone leaks and embolisms.

Scrotum—loose skin on a male that houses the testicles.

Seroma—a collection of fluid from blood (serum) that accumulates after a surgical operation or at a liposuction site.

Sex—male or female biologically. A female has an xx genotype and a male has an xy genotype. One can change one's external appearance to look like the opposite sex by having gender reassignment surgery but the original genotype will remain what the person was born with.

SGAP—this acronym stands for superior gluteal artery perforator flap. It is used to reconstruct a breast with tissue from the buttock. It was developed in 1993 by Robert Allen and Charles Tucker on a 28-year-old patient at Charity Hospital in New Orleans, Louisiana.

Silicone—a naturally occurring element that has been used for the majority of plastic surgery implants. Silicone-filled breast implants have largely been replaced with saline filled breast implants but the shell is still made from silicone.

Skin graft—a procedure where skin is taken from one part of the body and put on a part that was either removed because of skin cancer, trauma, burn or surgery.

Skin resurfacing—a variety of techniques such as dermabrasion to improve the overall appearance of the skin.

Soft tissue augmentation—the technique of filling defects with injectables such as collagen or hyaluronic acid.

Stahl's ear—an ear that has an abnormally shaped fold of cartilage.

Subsurface augmentation—This is a type of surgery used to fill out a defect, smooth out a contour or expand the skin that covers an area. Some implant materials are liquid, semisolid, powder, gel, liquid filled or gel filled, mesh, sheet or solid. There are natural implant materials from animals, from other parts of the patient's body or from another human. Natural materials used for subsurface augmentation are bone, cartilage, fascia, fat, ligament, membrane and skin. Synthetic materials are acrylic, adhesives, bioactive glass, ceramic, metal, plastics, silicone, and Teflon.

Suction lipectomy—liposuction.

Suprapubic—above the pubic bone, part of the pelvis below the navel.

Surgery—an invasive procedure which usually results in return or restoration of function or improvement in appearance.

Sutures—stitches.

Syndactyly—a genetic anomaly where fingers or toes are fused.

The Swan—a former reality Fox TV program that changed contestants from "ugly" to "beautiful" with a variety of procedures: plastic surgery, orthodontics, maxillofacial surgery, hair style and makeup.

Tendon—the white fibrous connective tissue that connects a muscle with a bone.

Tenolysis—surgery to separate a tendon from surrounding adhesions.

Thigh lift—the lateral (outer) and medial (inner) portions of the thigh that are flabby are targeted with incisions that cut from the outside of the thigh to the inside. Liposuction is combined with skin removal. Like the upper arm lift, a scar will remain.

Tissue expander—this is a device that it put under the skin to stretch it gradually so that it will accommodate whatever is underneath. Tissue expanders are used when there is not enough skin to cover the newly implanted device or when a wound is too large to be closed. Tissue expanders can be used in certain circumstances instead of skin grafts.

TRAM flap—a type of flap used to reconstruct a breast after it has been removed after a radical mastectomy. The acronym, TRAM, stands for transverse rectus abdominus musculocutaneous.

Transsexual—a gender orientation that a person switches by undergoing plastic surgery and extensive counseling to become the opposite gender.

Trigger finger—a condition where the finger snaps into place involuntarily. Plastic surgeons are qualified to perform hand surgery as well as other types of restorative, reparative and cosmetic surgery.

Tumescent liposuction—liposuction that is performed with an infusion of saline, epinephrine and Lidocaine prior to the fat removal.

Tummy tuck—abdominoplasty.

Ultrasound assisted lipoplasty—a type of liposuction that employs high frequency sound waves to liquefy the fat before it is sucked out.

Unilateral—one sided.

Upper arm lift—this surgery is for flabby skin under the arms. There are three techniques used: liposuction, surgical removal of excess skin and a combination of the two. The incision is made on the inside of the arm from the elbow to the armpit but since is so large, a scar will remain.

Varicose veins—veins that are abnormally swollen or dilated. They are visible under the skin, dark blue in color.

Venous system—the system of blood vessels that brings blood back to the heart.

Vitiligo—a condition where a normally dark skinned individual will have white patches of skin.

Z-plasty—a type of surgical incision that creates small triangular flaps to close wounds in places of the body where joints or bending occurs. A z-plasty scar revision creates those triangular flaps on the site of an original scar that repositions or changes the scar direction. It interrupts the tension that the scar puts on the skin and improves the flexibility of the tissue in the area.

Zerona—the brand name for a process that breaks down fat non surgically. The process involves a "cold" laser manufactured by Erchonia

NOTE

1. Jolly-Thorek, Thorek (2 types), Kuster, Kelly, Weinhold, Flesch, Thebesius and Weinscheimer, Schenelmann (four types), Eitner, Spaulding, Depage, and Babcock.

Further Reading

"Arthritis: Biologics Block Cytokines, Joint Replacement." eNotAlone. http://www.enotalone.com/article/7902.html.

Aufricht, Gustave. "The Development of Plastic Surgery in the United States." *Plastic and Reconstructive Surgery* 1 (1946): 25.

Bettmann, Otto. *A Pictorial History of Medicine.* Springfield, MO: Charles C. Thomas, 1972.

Bridges, Andrew. "Silicone Breast Implant Ban Lifted after 14 Years." http://www.chron.com/disp/story.mpl/business/4343687.html.

Carpue, J. C. *An Account of two successful operations for restoring a lost nose from the integuments of the forehead, in the cases of two officers of his majesty's army; to which are prefixed, historical and physiological remarks on the nasal operation; including descriptions of the Indian and Italian methods.* London: Longman, Hurst, Rees, Orme and Brown, 1816.

Celsus, Aulus Cornelius. *Celsus de Medicine with an English translation by W.G. Spencer in three Volumes.* London: William Heinemann, 1948. (Reprint of 1935 edition.)

Celsus, Aulus Cornelius. *De re medicina libri octo brevioribus.* Amstelaedami: Apud Joannem Wolters, 1687.

Flatt, A. E. "The Considered Use of Digital Joint Prostheses." In *Transactions of the Fifth International Congress of Plastic and Reconstructive Surgery.* Edited by J. T. Hueston, 638–48. Melbourne: Butterworths, 1971.

Fomon, Samuel. *Cosmetic Surgery: Principles and Practice.* Philadelphia: Lippincott, 1960.

Gilman, Sander. *Creating Beauty to Cure the Soul.* Durham, NC: Duke University Press, 1998.

Gilman, Sander. "Decircumcision: The First Aesthetic Surgery." *Modern Judaism* 17 (1997): 201–10.

Gilman, Sander. *Making the Body Beautiful: A Cultural History of Esthetic Surgery.* Princeton, NJ: Princeton University Press, 1999.

Gnudi, Martha Teach. *The Life and Times of Gaspare Tagliacozzi, Surgeon of Bologna, 1545–1599. With a Documented Study of the Scientific and Cultural Life of Bologna in the Sixteenth Century.* New York: Herbert Reichner, 1950.

Gould, Steven. *The Mismeasure of Man.* New York: W.W. Norton and Company, 1981.

Grealy, Lucy. *Autobiography of a Face.* Boston: Houghton Mifflin, 1994.

Haeger, Knut. *The Illustrated History of Surgery.* New York: Bell Publishing Company, 1988.

Haiken, Elizabeth. *Venus Envy: History of Cosmetic Surgery.* Baltimore: Johns Hopkins Press, 1997.

Holden, Harold M. *Noses.* Cleveland: The World Publishing Company, 1950.

Jugan, Milan J. "Liposculpting Procedures." In *Peterson's Principles of Oral and Maxillofacial Surgery,* ed. M. Miloro, 1407–18. Philadelphia: B.C. Decker, 2004.

Knapp, Arnold. "Victor Morax." *Archives of Ophthalmology* 14, no. 4 (1935): 641.

Lascaratos, John, Mimis Cohen, and Dionyssios Voros. "Plastic Surgery of the Face in Byzantium in the Fourth Century." *Plastic and Reconstructive Surgery* 106, no. 2 (2000): 1274–80.

Lucas, G.H.W., and V. E. Henderson. "A New Anesthetic: Cyclopropane." *Canadian Medical Association Journal* 21 (1929): 173–75.

Lyons, Albert S., and R. Joseph Petrucelli, II. *Medicine, an Illustrated History.* New York: Harry N. Abrams, 1987.

Man, Daniel. *The Art of Man: Faces of Plastic Surgery.* Boca Raton, FL: Beauty Arts Press, 1992.

Money, John. *Lovemaps.* New York: Irvington Publishers, 1986.

Morris, Desmond. *Manwatching.* New York: Harry N. Abrams, 1977.

Mutter, Thomas D. *Cases of Deformity from Burns, Successfully Treated by Plastic Operations.* Philadelphia: Merrihew and Thompson, 1843.

Owen, Edmund. *Cleft-Palate and Hare-Lip: The Earlier Operation on the Palate.* London: Baillière, Tindall and Cox, 1904.

Paré, Ambröise. *On Monsters and Marvels.* Translated with an introduction and notes by Janis L. Pallister. Chicago: The University of Chicago Press, 1982. (Based on the 1840 translation.)

Pollet, J., and J. Pillet. "Profileplasty-Forehead Silicone Implants." In *Transactions of the Fifth International Congress of Plastic and Reconstructive Surgery.* Edited by J.T. Hueston, 1136–40. Melbourne: Butterworths, 1971.

Price, Eroston, Harold Schueler, and Joshua Perper. "Massive Systemic Silicone Embolism: A Case Report and Review of Literature." *American Journal of Forensic Medicine and Pathology* 27, no. 2 (2006): 97–102.

Rittersma, Jan. "The Dentist as Plastic Surgeon (Hugo Ganzer 1879–1960)." *Journal of Cranio-Maxillo-Facial Surgery* 16 (1988): 51–54.

Santoni-Rugiu, Paolo, and R. Mazzola. "The Italian Contribution to Facial Plastic Surgery: A Historical Reappraisal." *Plastic and Reconstructive Surgery* 99 (1997): 570–75.

Santoni-Rugiu, Paolo, and Phillip Sykes. *A History of Plastic Surgery.* New York: Springer Verlag, 2007.

Skoog, Tord. *Plastic Surgery: New Methods and Refinements.* Stockholm: Almqvist and Wiksel International, 1974.

Sorta-Bilajac, Iva, and Amir Mazur. "The Nose between Ethics and Aesthetics: Sushruta's Legacy." *Otolaryngology—Head and Neck Surgery* 137 (2007): 707–10.

Stewart, Mary. *Silicone Spills: Breast Implants on Trial.* Westport, CT: Praeger, 1998.

Swanson, A.B. "A Silicone Rubber Implant for Resection Arthoplasty in the Hand." In *Transactions of the Fifth International Congress of Plastic and Reconstructive Surgery.* Edited by J.T. Hueston, 649–50. Melbourne: Butterworths, 1971.

Weimer, D. Robert. "The History and Development of the Breast Implant." http://breastimplants411.com/dbii/articles.asp~Article_ID=70.

Whitaker, Iain S., Richard O. Karoo, George Spyrou, and Oliver M. Fenton. "The Birth of Plastic Surgery: The Story of Nasal Reconstruction from the Edwin Smith Papyrus to the Twenty-first Century." *Plastic and Reconstructive Surgery* 120 (2007): 327–36.

Yalom, Marilyn. *A History of the Breast.* New York: Ballentine, 1997.

INDEX

ABOUT THE AUTHOR

Lana Thompson is an independent scholar who lives in Boca Raton, Florida, a community with an abundance of plastic surgeons and women who have chosen to have extreme body modifications with tummy tucks, breast augmentation, and Botox injections. She volunteers at the Broward County Medical Examiner's office in the morgue where the fatal downside of glamour arrives when plastic surgery goes wrong.

She has an MA in anthropology and an MFA in creative nonfiction. Her previous works include *The Wandering Womb: A Cultural History of Outrageous Beliefs about Women* and encyclopedia articles for medical, anthropological, and scientific venues. She is currently working on an *Encyclopedia of Death, Dying and Display of the Body* and an article about the relationship of cats with people.

DATE DUE
